COOKBOOK FOR HEALTHY RECIPES

The Complete Guide To Make Fast, Easy And Delicious Meals For Optimal Health

Dr Isabella Del Gusto

Copyright © 2024 Dr Isabella Del Gusto

TABLE OF CONTENT

INTRODUCTION

In the vibrant tapestry of life, the essence of true richness lies not in material possessions, but in the nourishment we provide our bodies and souls. Picture a lush garden, where every seed sown sprouts into a flourishing bouquet of vitality and joy. This is the realm of healthy eating, where the colors of nature's bounty dance on our plates, weaving a symphony of flavor and wellness.

In the heart of this garden, lies the profound importance of choosing wholesome foods over the allure of instant gratification offered by junk fare. It's a journey of love and care, where each bite becomes a brushstroke painting the canvas of our well-being. Like a cherished romance, the bond between nutritious meals and our bodies blossoms into a tale of longevity and contentment.

As we traverse this path, guided by the wisdom of generations past, we unearth treasures far beyond the reach of fleeting indulgences. The bounty of fruits, vegetables, and whole grains becomes the cornerstone of our vitality, nurturing not just our physical selves but also nurturing the bonds of family and community.

In this narrative of nourishment, every meal shared becomes a celebration of life, a testament to the joy found in embracing the gifts of nature. With each wholesome bite, we cultivate not just our bodies, but a legacy of well-being that resonates through the ages.

So let us embark on this odyssey of health, guided by the warmth of love and the promise of happiness. For in the garden of life, the seeds we sow today shall blossom into the bountiful harvest of tomorrow, where richness is measured not by what we possess, but by the vitality that thrives within us.

Importance of Healthy Eating:

Healthy eating plays a pivotal role in maintaining overall well-being and preventing various health issues. It encompasses consuming a balanced diet rich in essential nutrients, vitamins, and minerals while avoiding excessive intake of unhealthy foods.

- Nutrient Supply: A healthy diet provides the body with the necessary nutrients it needs to function optimally. These nutrients include carbohydrates, proteins, fats, vitamins, minerals, and water, which are vital for energy production, tissue repair, immune function, and various metabolic processes.

- Weight Management: Adopting a healthy eating pattern can help in managing body weight effectively. Consuming a diet that is high in fruits, vegetables, whole grains, and lean proteins, while limiting the intake of processed foods and sugary beverages, can contribute to weight control and reduce the risk of obesity-related complications.

- Disease Prevention: Healthy eating habits are associated with a reduced risk of chronic diseases such as heart disease, diabetes, hypertension, and certain types of cancer. A diet rich in fruits, vegetables, whole grains, and healthy fats can help lower cholesterol levels, regulate blood sugar levels, and maintain blood pressure within a healthy range.

- Enhanced Mental Health: There is growing evidence to suggest that a balanced diet can positively impact mental health and cognitive function. Nutrient-rich foods, such as fatty fish, nuts, seeds, and leafy greens, contain compounds that support brain health and may help reduce the risk of depression, anxiety, and age-related cognitive decline.

- Improved Digestion: Fiber-rich foods, such as fruits, vegetables, whole grains, and legumes, promote digestive health by regulating bowel movements, preventing constipation, and supporting the growth of beneficial gut bacteria. A healthy digestive system is essential for nutrient absorption and overall vitality.

- Increased Energy Levels: Consuming a diet that is nutritionally balanced and provides adequate calories can help sustain energy levels throughout the day. By fueling the body with wholesome foods and avoiding excessive consumption of processed foods and refined sugars, individuals can experience improved stamina and productivity.

The Importance of Occasional Fasting for Health:

While healthy eating is essential for overall well-being, occasional fasting or controlled periods of food restriction can also offer health benefits. Here's why intermittent fasting or occasional fasting can be advantageous:

- Improved Metabolic Health: Fasting intermittently can help regulate insulin sensitivity, promote fat metabolism, and enhance cellular repair processes. It may also contribute to weight loss and reduce the risk of metabolic disorders such as type 2 diabetes and insulin resistance.
- Cellular Repair and Autophagy: Fasting triggers autophagy, a cellular process that involves the removal of damaged or dysfunctional components within cells. This mechanism helps rejuvenate cells, promote longevity, and may reduce the risk of age-related diseases.
- Enhanced Brain Function: Some research suggests that intermittent fasting may have neuroprotective effects and promote brain health by increasing the production of brain-derived neurotrophic factor (BDNF), a protein that supports neuronal growth and cognitive function.
- Inflammation Reduction: Fasting has been shown to decrease markers of inflammation in the body, which is associated with a reduced risk of chronic diseases such as heart disease, arthritis, and certain types of cancer.
- Promotes Mindful Eating: Intermittent fasting encourages individuals to be more mindful of their eating habits and food choices. By restricting the window of food consumption, individuals may become more attuned to hunger cues and develop a healthier relationship with food.

Tips for Healthy Cooking and Eating

Cooking and eating healthily are essential components of maintaining overall well-being and preventing chronic diseases. By incorporating nutritious ingredients and mindful cooking techniques, individuals can optimize their health and enjoy delicious meals.

Prioritize Whole Foods:

- Pick complete, unprocessed foods including vegetables, fruits, whole grains, lean meats, and healthy fats.
- Incorporate a variety of colorful fruits and vegetables into meals to ensure a diverse range of vitamins, minerals, and antioxidants.

Limit Processed Foods:

- Minimize the consumption of processed foods that are high in added sugars, unhealthy fats, sodium, and preservatives.
- Read food labels carefully and opt for products with minimal ingredients and no artificial additives.

Opt for Healthy Cooking Methods:

- Use cooking methods such as steaming, grilling, baking, roasting, and sautéing instead of frying or deep-frying to reduce the amount of added fats.

- Experiment with herbs, spices, and citrus juices to enhance flavor without relying on excessive salt or sugar.

Control Portion Sizes:

- Be mindful of portion sizes to avoid overeating and unnecessary calorie intake.
- Use smaller plates and bowls to help manage portion sizes and prevent overindulgence.

Include Lean Proteins:

- Incorporate lean protein sources such as skinless poultry, fish, tofu, legumes, and beans into meals to support muscle growth, repair, and satiety.
- Limit the consumption of red and processed meats, which are associated with an increased risk of heart disease and certain cancers.

Choose Healthy Fats:

- Opt for sources of healthy fats such as avocados, nuts, seeds, olive oil, and fatty fish rich in omega-3 fatty acids.

- Reduce your consumption of baked goods, processed snacks, and fried foods that contain saturated and trans fats.

Be Mindful of Added Sugars:

- Reduce the consumption of sugary beverages, desserts, and snacks by choosing naturally sweetened options or homemade alternatives.

- Use natural sweeteners like honey, maple syrup, or dates in moderation when necessary.

Stay Hydrated:

- Drink an adequate amount of water throughout the day to maintain hydration and support proper bodily functions.
- Limit the consumption of sugary drinks and opt for water, herbal teas, or infused water with fresh fruits and herbs.

Plan and Prepare Meals:

- Plan meals ahead of time to ensure balanced nutrition and avoid relying on unhealthy convenience foods.
- Prep ingredients in advance, such as washing and chopping fruits and vegetables, to streamline cooking and make healthy choices more accessible.

Practice Mindful Eating:

- Slow down and savor each bite by chewing food thoroughly and paying attention to hunger and fullness cues.
- Avoid distractions such as television or electronic devices during meals to promote mindful eating and prevent overeating.

1

Breakfast Recipes

Green Smoothie Bowl

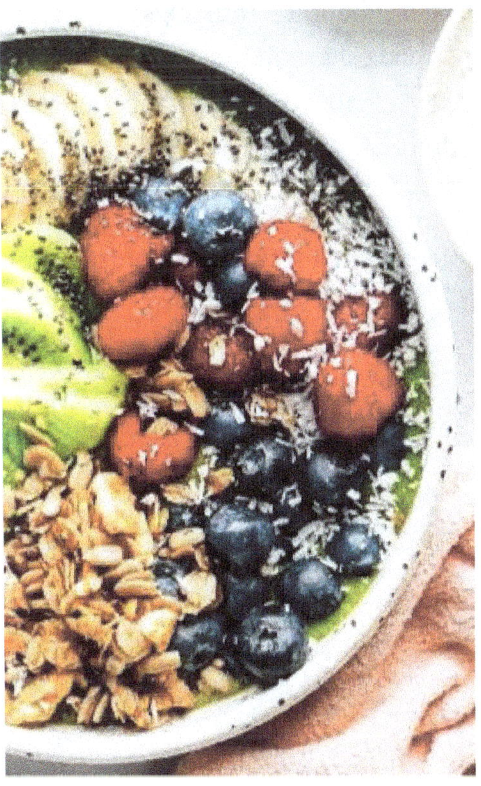

Time of Preparation:

- Total time: 10 minutes

Ingredients:

- 2 ripe bananas, frozen and sliced
- 1 cup fresh spinach leaves
- 1/2 avocado, peeled and pitted
- 1/2 cup plain Greek yogurt
- Half a cup of almond milk, or any other type of milk.
- 1 tablespoon honey or maple syrup (optional, for sweetness)
- Toppings (optional): sliced fruits (such as berries, kiwi, or mango), granola, chia seeds, shredded coconut, nuts, or seeds

Procedure:

- In a blender, combine the frozen bananas, spinach leaves, avocado, Greek yogurt, almond milk, and honey (if using).
- Blend until smooth and creamy, stopping the blender occasionally to scrape down the sides to make sure all of the ingredients are completely combined.
- Pour the smoothie into bowls.
- Top with your favorite toppings, such as sliced fruits, granola, chia seeds, shredded coconut, nuts, or seeds.
- Serve immediately and enjoy!

Tips and Tricks:

- Use ripe bananas for natural sweetness and creamy texture.
- Freeze the bananas in advance to make the smoothie cold and creamy without needing ice cubes.
- Experiment with different combinations of fruits and greens to vary the flavor and nutritional content.
- Adjust the consistency of the smoothie by adding more or less almond milk.
- For an additional taste and protein boost, add nut butter or protein powder.

Nutritional Value per Serving:

- **Calories: approximately 250 kcal**
- **Protein: 8g**

- **Fat: 10g**
- **Carbohydrates: 35g**
- **Fiber: 7g**
- **Sugar: 20g**

Caution and Precautions:

- If you have allergies to any of the ingredients, please avoid or substitute accordingly.
- Be cautious when using a blender and handling sharp objects.
- Make sure all fruits and vegetables are properly washed before use.

Healthy Additions:

- Add a handful of kale or Swiss chard for additional nutrients.
- Incorporate a tablespoon of ground flaxseeds or hemp seeds for omega-3 fatty acids.
- Include a scoop of plant-based protein powder for added protein content.

Health Benefits

- Packed with vitamins, minerals, and antioxidants from spinach, avocado, and fruits.
- Rich in fiber, which supports gut health and facilitates digestion.
- Contains healthy fats from avocado, which are beneficial for heart health.
- Provides a good source of protein and energy for a satisfying breakfast or snack.

Safety Measures

- Wash hands thoroughly before handling ingredients.
- Use clean utensils and kitchen equipment.
- Remaining food can be kept in the refrigerator for up to 24 hours if it is sealed tightly.

Avocado Toast with Poached Egg

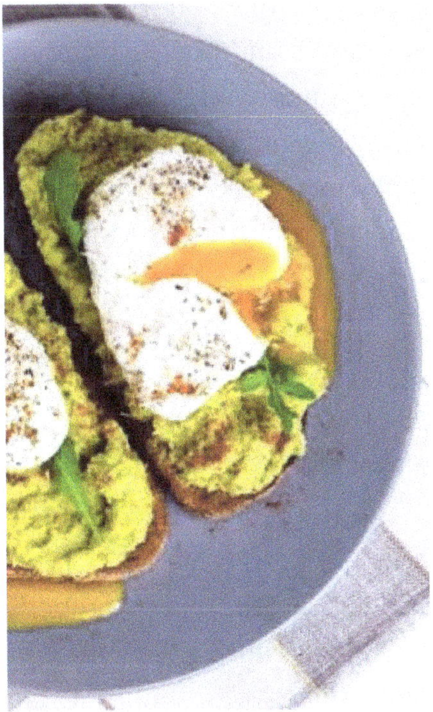

Time of Preparation:

- Total time: 15 minutes

Ingredients:

- 2 ripe avocados
- 4 slices of whole grain bread
- 4 large eggs
- Salt and pepper to taste
- Optional toppings: sliced tomatoes, microgreens, red pepper flakes, or hot sauce

Procedure:

- Remove the pits from the avocados, cut them in half, and scoop out the meat into a bowl.
- Mash the avocado with a fork until smooth but still slightly chunky.

- Toast the whole grain bread slices till crispy and golden brown.
- While the bread is toasting, fill a medium-sized saucepan with water and bring it to a gentle simmer.

- Crack each egg into a ramekin or small basin.
- Carefully slide the eggs, one at a time, into the simmering water. Poach the eggs for 3-4 minutes until the whites are set but the yolks are still runny.
- Using a slotted spoon, remove the poached eggs from the water and place them on a paper towel to drain excess water.

- Gently place each egg into the simmering water one at a time.
- To taste, add salt and pepper to the avocado.
- Top each avocado toast with a poached egg.
- Garnish with optional toppings like sliced tomatoes, microgreens, red pepper flakes, or hot sauce.
- Serve immediately and enjoy!

Tips and Tricks:

- Choose ripe avocados for optimal flavor and creamy texture.

- To get more minerals and fiber, use whole grain bread.
- Squeeze in some lemon or lime juice into the mashed avocado to keep it from browning.

- For perfectly poached eggs, use fresh eggs and ensure the water is gently simmering, not boiling vigorously.
- Use a slotted spoon to remove the poached eggs from the water to drain excess liquid.

Nutritional Value per Serving:

- **Calories: approximately 300 kcal**
- **Protein: 15g**
- **Fat: 20g**
- **Carbohydrates: 20g**
- **Fiber: 8g**
- **Sugar: 2g**

Caution and Precautions:

- Be cautious when handling hot water and poaching eggs to prevent burns.
- Ensure eggs are cooked thoroughly before consuming.
- If you have allergies to any of the ingredients, please avoid or substitute accordingly.

Healthy Additions:

- Add a sprinkle of nutritional yeast or feta cheese for extra flavor.
- Include sliced smoked salmon or turkey bacon for added protein and flavor.

Health Benefits

- Avocado provides healthy fats, fiber, and essential nutrients like potassium and vitamins.
- Whole grain bread offers complex carbohydrates and fiber, which aids digestion and promotes satiety.
- Eggs are rich in protein, vitamins, and minerals, including vitamin D and choline, which are essential for brain health.

Safety Measures

- Wash hands thoroughly before handling food.
- Use clean utensils and kitchen surfaces.
- Ensure eggs are fresh and properly cooked to reduce the risk of foodborne illness.

Quinoa Breakfast Bowl

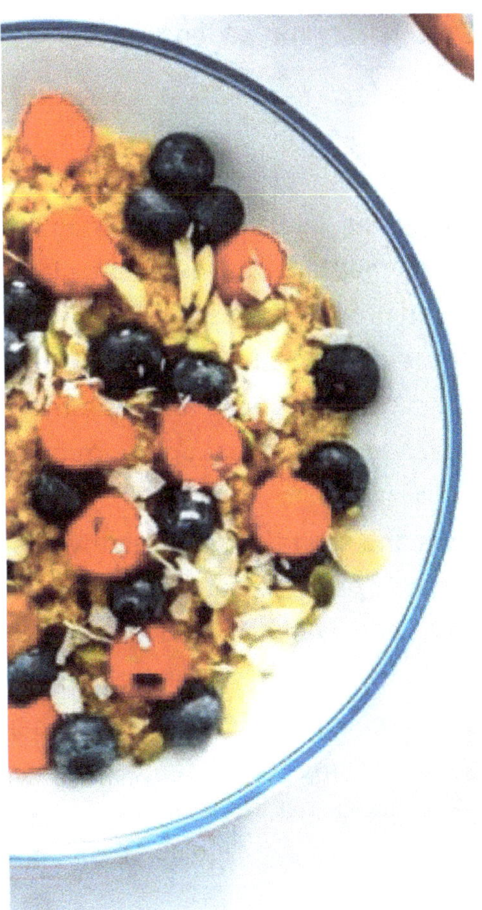

Time of Preparation:

- Total time: 25 minutes

Ingredients:

- 1/2 cup quinoa, rinsed
- 1 cup water or vegetable broth
- 1 ripe banana, sliced
- 1/2 cup fresh berries (such as strawberries, blueberries, or raspberries)
- 2 tablespoons nuts or seeds (such as almonds, walnuts, pumpkin seeds, or chia seeds)
- 1 tablespoon honey or maple syrup (optional, for sweetness)
- 1/2 teaspoon cinnamon (optional, for flavor)
- Optional toppings: sliced fruits, shredded coconut, nut butter, yogurt, or granola

Procedure:

- In a small saucepan, combine the quinoa and water or vegetable broth. Bring to a boil, then reduce heat to low, cover, and simmer for 15-20 minutes, or until the quinoa is cooked and the liquid is absorbed.
- Fluff the cooked quinoa with a fork and divide it evenly into two bowls.
- Arrange the sliced banana, fresh berries, and nuts or seeds on top of the quinoa.
- Drizzle with honey or maple syrup and sprinkle with cinnamon, if desired.
- Add any optional toppings of your choice, such as sliced fruits, shredded coconut, nut butter, yogurt, or granola.
- Serve warm and enjoy!

Tips and Tricks:

- To get rid of any bitterness, rinse the quinoa under cold water before cooking.
- Use a 2:1 ratio of water to quinoa for optimal cooking results.
- Customize the toppings to your preference and dietary needs.

- Cook a larger batch of quinoa ahead of time and store it in the refrigerator for quick and easy breakfast bowls throughout the week.
- Experiment with different flavor combinations by adding spices like nutmeg or cardamom, or using alternative sweeteners like agave syrup or date syrup.

Nutritional Value per Serving:

- **Calories: approximately 300 kcal**
- **Protein: 8g**
- **Fat: 6g**
- **Carbohydrates: 55g**
- **Fiber: 8g**
- **Sugar: 15g**

Caution and Precautions:

- Be cautious when handling hot pots and pans during cooking.
- Check the quinoa for any debris or impurities before cooking.
- If you have allergies to any of the ingredients, please avoid or substitute accordingly.

Healthy Additions:

- Add a dollop of Greek yogurt or coconut yogurt for extra creaminess and probiotics.
- Incorporate chopped fruits like apples or pears for additional sweetness and fiber.
- Mix in a tablespoon of ground flaxseeds or hemp seeds for omega-3 fatty acids and added texture.

Health Benefits

- Quinoa is a complete protein, containing all nine essential amino acids, making it an excellent plant-based protein source.
- Berries are rich in antioxidants, vitamins, and fiber, which promote heart health and support immune function.
- Nuts and seeds provide healthy fats, protein, and essential nutrients, such as magnesium and zinc, which are important for overall well-being.
- This breakfast bowl is high in fiber and complex carbohydrates, providing sustained energy and promoting satiety throughout the morning.

Safety Measures

- Wash hands thoroughly before handling food.
- Ensure quinoa is cooked thoroughly to prevent foodborne illness.
- Any leftovers can be kept in the fridge for up to three days if they are kept in an airtight container.

2

Appetizers and Snacks

Greek Yogurt Veggie Dip

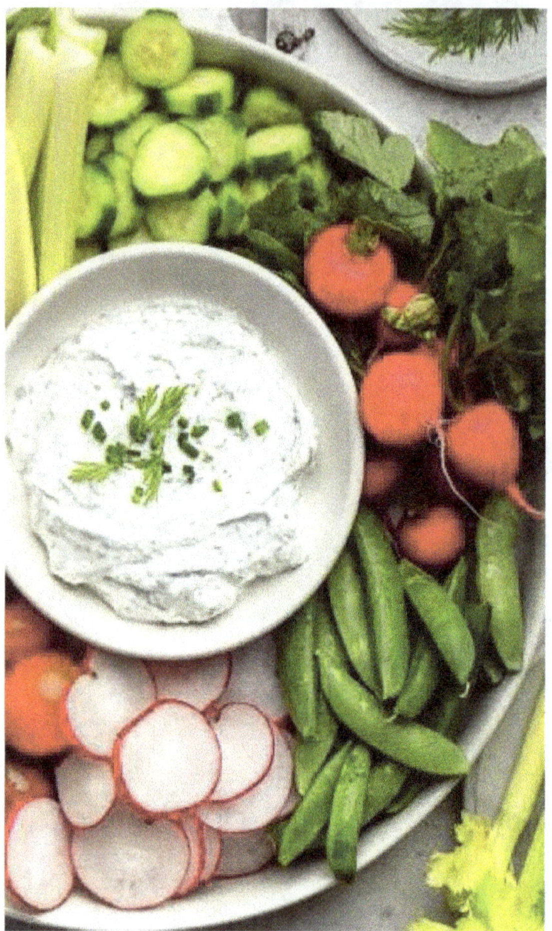

Time of Preparation:

- Approximately 10 minutes

Ingredients:

- 1 cup Greek yogurt
- 1/2 cup finely chopped cucumber
- 1/2 cup finely chopped red bell pepper
- 1/4 cup finely chopped red onion
- 2 cloves garlic, minced
- 2 tablespoons fresh lemon juice
- One tablespoon of freshly chopped dill (or one teaspoon of dried dill)
- Salt and pepper to taste

Procedure:

- In a mixing bowl, combine Greek yogurt, chopped cucumber, red bell pepper, red onion, minced garlic, lemon juice, and chopped dill.
- Stir the ingredients until well combined.
- Adjust the amount of salt and pepper to taste.
- To give the tastes time to mingle, cover the bowl and place it in the refrigerator for at least half an hour.
- Serve chilled with fresh cut vegetables, pita bread, or crackers.

Tips and Tricks:

- Use thick Greek yogurt for a creamier texture.
- Drain excess moisture from the cucumber before adding it to the dip to prevent it from becoming watery.
- Adjust the amount of garlic and lemon juice according to personal preference.
- Experiment with different herbs like mint or parsley for variation.

Nutritional Value per Serving (1/4 cup):

- Calories: 60
- Total Fat: 0.5g
- Cholesterol: 3mg
- Sodium: 25mg
- Carbohydrates: 7g
- Fiber: 1g

- **Sugars: 4g**
- **Protein: 7g**

Caution and Precautions:

- Ensure all vegetables are washed thoroughly before chopping.
- Store leftover dip in an airtight container in the refrigerator and consume within 2-3 days.
- Avoid leaving the dip at room temperature for an extended period to prevent bacterial growth.

Healthy Addition:

- Add grated carrots or chopped spinach for additional nutrients and color.

Health Benefits

- Greek yogurt is rich in protein, calcium, and probiotics which promote gut health and digestion.
- Vegetables like cucumber, red bell pepper, and onion provide vitamins, minerals, and antioxidants that support overall health.
- Garlic is known for its immune-boosting properties and may help lower cholesterol levels.

Safety Measures

- Wash hands thoroughly before handling food.

- Cut meat and vegetables on different cutting boards to avoid cross-contamination.

- Refrigerate perishable ingredients promptly to maintain freshness and prevent spoilage.
- Clean and sanitize kitchen surfaces and utensils regularly to minimize the risk of foodborne illness.

Baked Sweet Potato Fries

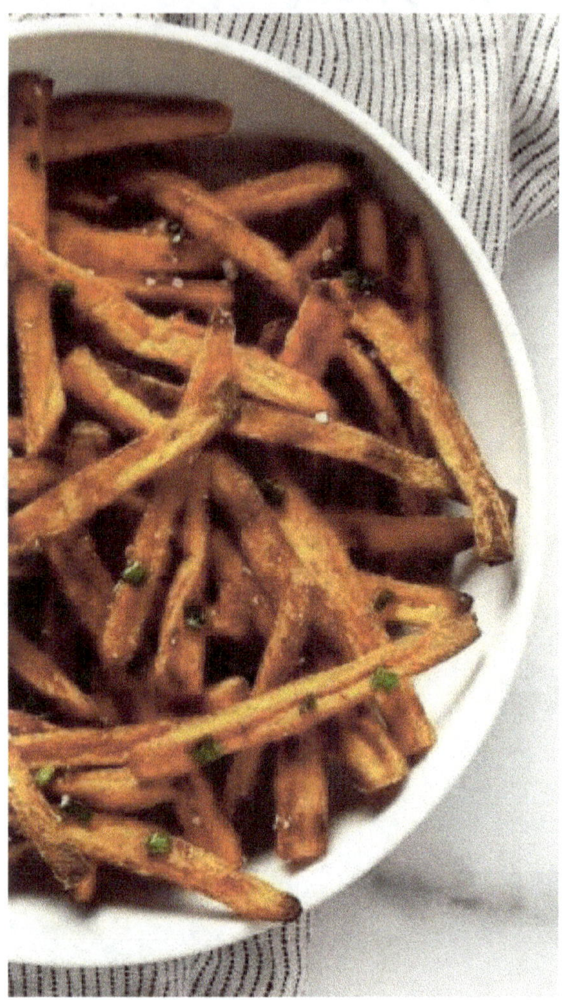

Time of Preparation:

- Approximately 30-35 minutes

Ingredients:

- Two big sweet potatoes, cleaned and de-seeded
- 2 tablespoons olive oil
- 1 teaspoon paprika
- 1/2 teaspoon garlic powder
- 1/2 teaspoon onion powder
- Salt and pepper to taste

- Optional: chopped fresh herbs like rosemary or thyme for garnish

Procedure:

- Preheat the oven to 425°F (220°C) and line a baking sheet with parchment paper or aluminum foil.
- Cut the sweet potatoes into uniform fries or wedges, about 1/4 to 1/2 inch thick.
- In a large bowl, toss the sweet potato fries with olive oil, paprika, garlic powder, onion powder, salt, and pepper until evenly coated.

- On the prepared baking sheet, arrange the fries in a single layer, taking care not to crowd them.
- Fries should be baked for 20 to 25 minutes in a preheated oven, turning them over halfway through, until they are crispy and golden brown.
- Once done, remove from the oven and sprinkle with additional salt and chopped fresh herbs if desired.
- Serve hot with your favorite dipping sauce.

Tips and Tricks:

- To guarantee equal baking, chop the sweet potatoes into uniform pieces.
- Soak the cut sweet potatoes in cold water for about 30 minutes before baking to remove excess starch, which helps achieve crispier fries.
- Place the fries in a single layer on the baking sheet to avoid

overcrowding, which can result in soggy fries.

- For extra crispiness, you can sprinkle a light coating of cornstarch on the fries before tossing them with olive oil and spices.

Nutritional Value per Serving (1/2 cup):

- **Calories: 120**
- **Total Fat: 4g**
- **Saturated Fat: 0.5g**
- **Sodium: 150mg**
- **Carbohydrates: 21g**
- **Fiber: 3g**
- **Sugars: 6g**
- **Protein: 2g**

Caution and Precautions:

- Use caution when cutting sweet potatoes to prevent injury.
- Be careful when handling hot baking sheets and oven racks.
- Ensure the sweet potatoes are thoroughly washed and peeled to remove any dirt or debris.

Healthy Addition:

- Serve with a side of Greek yogurt dip or hummus for added protein and flavor.
- Sprinkle nutritional yeast over the fries for a cheesy flavor without the added calories.

Health Benefits

- Sweet potatoes are a rich source of fiber, vitamins A and C, and potassium, which support immune function, vision health, and heart health.
- Baking the sweet potatoes instead of frying reduces the amount of added fat and calories, making this recipe a healthier alternative to traditional fries.
- Olive oil used in this recipe is high in monounsaturated fats, which can help lower bad cholesterol levels and reduce the risk of heart disease.

Safety Measures

- Wash hands thoroughly before handling food.
- Use a clean, sharp knife and cutting board to cut the sweet potatoes.
- Store leftover fries in an airtight container in the refrigerator and consume within 2-3 days.
- Clean and sanitize kitchen surfaces and utensils regularly to prevent cross-contamination.

Hummus with Crudites

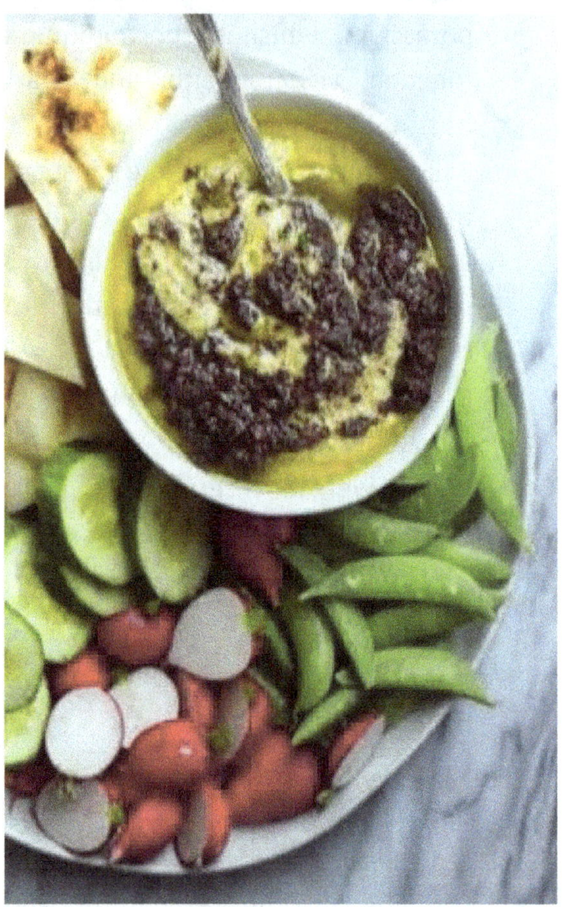

Time of Preparation:

- Approximately 15-20 minutes

Ingredients:

- **For Hummus:**

- One can (15 ounces) of rinsed and drained chickpeas
- 1/4 cup tahini
- 1/4 cup fresh lemon juice
- 2 cloves garlic, minced
- 2 tablespoons olive oil
- 1/2 teaspoon ground cumin
- Salt to taste

- Water (as needed for desired consistency)
- **For Crudites:**

- Assorted vegetables such as carrots, cucumbers, bell peppers, cherry tomatoes, and celery, washed and sliced

Procedure:

- In a food processor, combine the chickpeas, tahini, lemon juice, minced garlic, olive oil, ground cumin, and salt.

- Process until smooth, stopping occasionally to scrape down the bowl's sides.
- . If the hummus is too thick, add water, a tablespoon at a time, until the desired consistency is reached.
- Taste and adjust seasoning as necessary, adding more lemon juice, garlic, or salt according to your preference.

- After transferring the hummus to a serving bowl, pour in a small amount of additional olive oil. If preferred, garnish with chopped fresh herbs or a dash of paprika.
- Arrange the assorted vegetable crudites around the hummus bowl for dipping.

Tips and Tricks:

- For creamier hummus, remove the skins from the chickpeas before processing. Simply rub the chickpeas between your fingers under running water to loosen the skins, then discard them.

- Add a tablespoon of Greek yogurt for extra creaminess and tanginess.
- Experiment with different flavor variations by adding roasted red peppers, sun-dried tomatoes, or fresh herbs like parsley or cilantro to the hummus.
- To make the hummus ahead of time, store it in an airtight container in the refrigerator for up to a week.

Nutritional Value per Serving (2 tablespoons of hummus with assorted vegetables):

- **Calories: 70**
- **Total Fat: 5g**
- **Saturated Fat: 0.5g**
- **Sodium: 70mg**
- **Carbohydrates: 6g**
- **Fiber: 2g**
- **Sugars: 1g**
- **Protein: 2g**

Caution and Precautions:

- Be cautious when handling the blade of the food processor.
- Wash vegetables thoroughly before slicing and serving to remove any dirt or pesticides.
- Store leftover hummus and crudites in separate airtight containers in the refrigerator.

Healthy Addition:

- Sprinkle toasted sesame seeds or pine nuts on top of the hummus for added texture and flavor.
- Serve with whole grain pita bread or whole wheat crackers for a nutritious snack or appetizer.

Health Benefits

- Chickpeas are a good source of protein, fiber, and complex carbohydrates, which help promote satiety and stabilize blood sugar levels.

- Rich in calcium, iron, and magnesium, as well as good fats and vitamins, is tahini.
- Vegetables provide essential vitamins, minerals, and antioxidants that support overall health and immune function.
- Olive oil is high in monounsaturated fats, which have been shown to reduce the risk of heart disease and improve cholesterol levels.

Safety Measures

- Wash hands thoroughly before handling food.

- Cut meat and vegetables on different cutting boards to avoid cross-contamination.
- Refrigerate leftover hummus and crudites promptly to prevent bacterial growth.

- Clean and sanitize kitchen surfaces and utensils regularly to maintain a hygienic cooking environment.

3

Salad Creations

Kale and Quinoa Salad

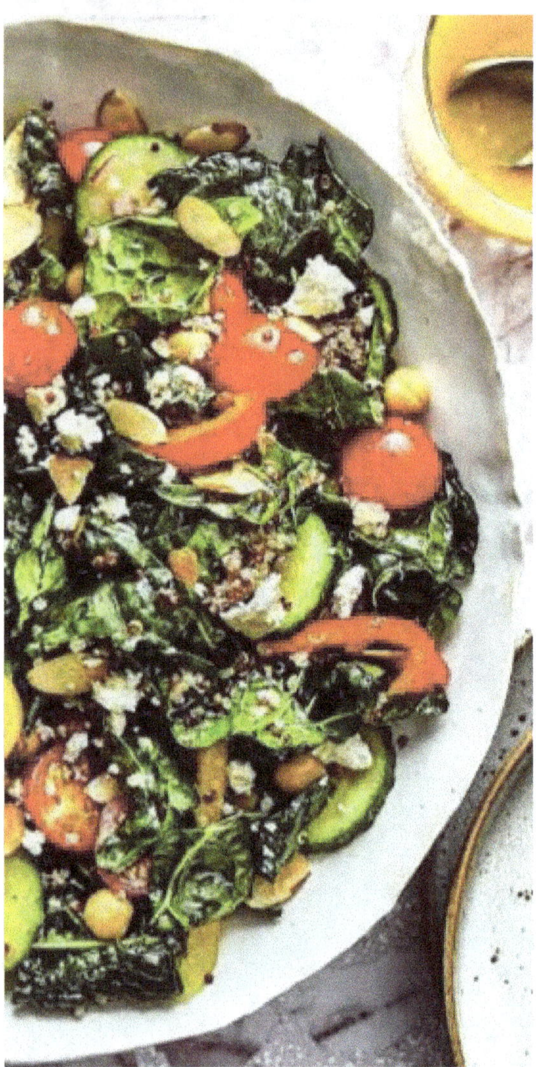

Time of Preparation:

- Approximately 30 minutes

Ingredients:

- 1 cup quinoa
- 2 cups water or vegetable broth
- 1 bunch kale, stems removed and leaves chopped
- 1/4 cup extra virgin olive oil
- 2 tablespoons lemon juice
- 2 cloves garlic, minced
- 1/4 teaspoon salt
- 1/4 teaspoon black pepper
- 1/4 cup dried cranberries
- 1/4 cup sliced almonds
- Optional: feta cheese or goat cheese for topping

Procedure:

- Using a fine-mesh strainer, thoroughly rinse the quinoa under cold water.
- Bring the vegetable broth or water to a boil in a medium saucepan. Add the quinoa, reduce heat to low, cover, and simmer for about 15 minutes or until the quinoa is tender and the liquid is absorbed.
- In a small bowl, whisk together the extra virgin olive oil, lemon juice, minced garlic, salt, and black pepper to make the dressing.
- In a large mixing bowl, combine the chopped kale with the dressing. Massage the kale with your hands for a few minutes to help soften it.
- After cooking, use a fork to fluff the quinoa and allow it to cool slightly.
- Add the cooked quinoa, dried cranberries, and sliced almonds to the bowl with the kale. Toss everything together until well combined.
- If desired, sprinkle feta cheese or goat cheese over the top of the salad before serving.

Tips and Tricks:

- Massaging the kale helps to break down its tough fibers and makes it more tender and flavorful.
- Toasting the almonds before adding them to the salad enhances their nutty flavor.
- For added sweetness and texture, you can also add diced apples or pears to the salad.

Nutritional Value per Serving:

- **Calories: approximately 300**
- **Protein: 8g**
- **Carbohydrates: 30g**
- **Fiber: 5g**
- **Fat: 18g**
- **Iron: 15% of the Daily Value**
- **Vitamin C: 90% of the Daily Value**
- **Calcium: 10% of the Daily Value**

Caution and Precautions:

- Be cautious when massaging the kale to avoid tearing or damaging the leaves.
- Ensure that the quinoa is cooked thoroughly to avoid any risk of foodborne illness.

Healthy Addition:

- Adding additional vegetables such as cherry tomatoes, cucumbers, or bell peppers can increase the nutrient content and add freshness to the salad.

Health Benefits

- Kale is rich in vitamins A, C, and K, as well as antioxidants and fiber, which can help support healthy digestion and immune function.

- Quinoa is a great option for vegetarians and vegans because it is a complete protein source that includes all nine essential amino acids.
- Olive oil provides heart-healthy monounsaturated fats and antioxidants, which may help reduce inflammation and lower the risk of chronic diseases.
- Cranberries are packed with vitamin C and antioxidants, which can help promote urinary tract health and protect against oxidative stress.

Safety Measures

- Wash all produce thoroughly before use to remove any dirt or contaminants.
- Use separate cutting boards and utensils for raw meat and vegetables to prevent cross-contamination.
- Store leftovers in an airtight container in the refrigerator for up to 3-4 days, and discard any leftovers that have been left out at room temperature for more than 2 hours.

Spinach and Strawberry Salad

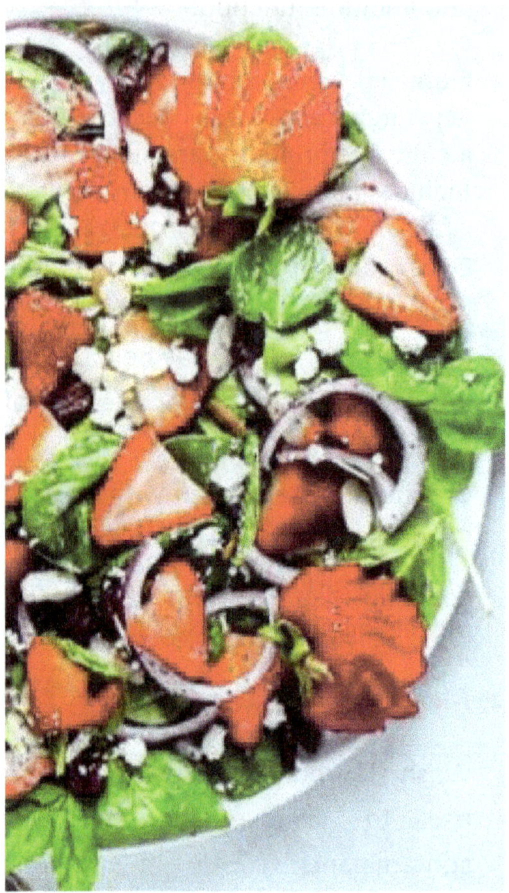

Time of Preparation:

- Approximately 20 minutes

Ingredients:

- 6 cups fresh baby spinach leaves

- One pint of freshly sliced and hulled strawberries
- 1/4 cup sliced almonds, toasted

- 1/4 cup of optionally shredded goat or feta cheese

- 1/4 cup balsamic vinegar
- 2 tablespoons extra virgin olive oil
- 1 tablespoon honey
- Salt and pepper to taste

Procedure:

- Sliced strawberries and fresh baby spinach leaves should be combined in a big mixing dish.
- In a small bowl, whisk together the balsamic vinegar, extra virgin olive oil, honey, salt, and pepper to make the dressing.
- Pour the dressing over the spinach and strawberry mixture and toss gently to coat.
- Sprinkle the toasted sliced almonds and crumbled feta cheese or goat cheese over the top of the salad.
- Serve immediately and enjoy!

Tips and Tricks:

- Toasting the sliced almonds adds depth of flavor and crunch to the salad. To toast almonds, spread them evenly on a baking sheet and bake in a preheated oven at 350°F (175°C) for 5-7 minutes, or until lightly golden brown.
- Choose ripe strawberries for the best flavor and sweetness.
- You can also add thinly sliced red onions or avocado for additional flavor and texture.

Nutritional Value per Serving:

- **Calories: approximately 150**

- **Protein: 4g**
- **Carbohydrates: 12g**
- **Fiber: 4g**
- **Fat: 10g**
- **Vitamin C: 90% of the Daily Value**
- **Vitamin A: 110% of the Daily Value**
- **Calcium: 10% of the Daily Value**
- **Iron: 15% of the Daily Value**

Caution and Precautions:

- Ensure that the spinach and strawberries are thoroughly washed before use to remove any dirt or contaminants.
- If you have nut allergies, omit the sliced almonds or substitute with toasted pumpkin seeds or sunflower seeds.

Healthy Addition:

- Adding grilled chicken breast or tofu can increase the protein content of the salad and make it a more filling meal option.

Health Benefits

- Spinach is a nutrient-dense leafy green vegetable that is rich in vitamins A, C, and K, as well as iron, calcium, and antioxidants, which can help support overall health and wellbeing.
- Strawberries are packed with vitamin C, fiber, and antioxidants, which can help boost immune function, promote heart health, and protect against chronic diseases.
- Olive oil provides heart-healthy monounsaturated fats and antioxidants, while honey adds natural sweetness without the need for refined sugars.

Safety Measures

- Wash your hands thoroughly before handling any fresh produce or ingredients.
- Use separate cutting boards and utensils for raw meat and vegetables to prevent cross-contamination.
- Store leftovers in an airtight container in the refrigerator for up to 2-3 days, and discard any leftovers that have been left out at room temperature for more than 2 hours.

Mediterranean Chickpea Salad

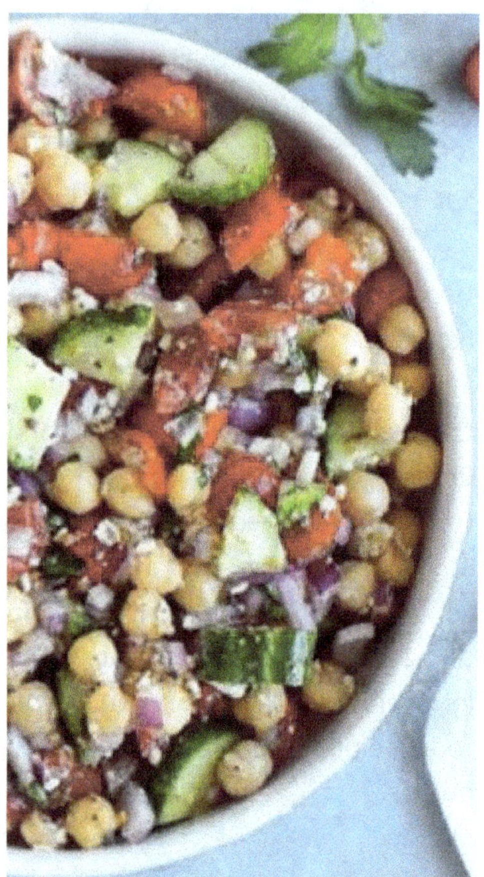

Time of Preparation:

- Approximately 25 minutes

Ingredients:

- Two cans of washed and drained chickpeas, 15 ounces each
- 1 English cucumber, diced
- 1 pint cherry tomatoes, halved
- 1/2 red onion, finely diced
- 1/2 cup Kalamata olives, pitted and sliced
- 1/2 cup crumbled feta cheese
- 1/4 cup fresh parsley, chopped
- 1/4 cup extra virgin olive oil
- 2 tablespoons red wine vinegar
- 1 teaspoon dried oregano
- Salt and pepper to taste

Procedure:

- Chickpeas, diced cucumber, diced red onion, split cherry tomatoes, sliced Kalamata olives, crumbled feta cheese, and chopped parsley should all be combined in a big mixing basin.
- To make the dressing, combine the dried oregano, extra virgin olive oil, red wine vinegar, salt, and pepper in a small bowl.
- After adding the dressing, gently toss to coat the chickpea salad.
- Taste and adjust seasoning, if necessary.
- Serve immediately or refrigerate for at least 30 minutes to allow the flavors to meld before serving.

Tips and Tricks:

- For extra flavor, you can roast the chickpeas in the oven with a drizzle of olive oil and your favorite seasonings before adding them to the salad.
- If you prefer a milder onion flavor, soak the diced red onion in cold water for 10-15 minutes before adding it to the salad.
- Use fresh herbs like mint or basil for added freshness and aroma.

Nutritional Value per Serving:

- **Calories: approximately 250**
- **Protein: 10g**
- **Carbohydrates: 25g**
- **Fiber: 6g**
- **Fat: 14g**
- **Vitamin C: 25% of the Daily Value**
- **Iron: 15% of the Daily Value**
- **Calcium: 15% of the Daily Value**

Caution and Precautions:

- Check the labels of canned chickpeas and olives for added salt or preservatives, and choose low-sodium options whenever possible.
- If you have a dairy allergy or follow a vegan diet, omit the feta cheese or substitute with a dairy-free alternative.

Healthy Addition:

- Adding diced avocado or roasted red peppers can enhance the flavor and nutritional value of the salad.

Health Benefits

- Chickpeas are a good source of plant-based protein, fiber, and complex carbohydrates, which can help regulate blood sugar levels, promote digestive health, and support weight management.
- Olive oil provides heart-healthy monounsaturated fats and antioxidants, which may help reduce inflammation and lower the risk of chronic diseases.
- Tomatoes are rich in vitamins A and C, as well as antioxidants like lycopene, which can help protect against oxidative stress and reduce the risk of certain cancers.

Safety Measures

- Rinse all canned ingredients thoroughly under cold water to remove excess sodium and preservatives.
- Store leftovers in an airtight container in the refrigerator for up to 3-4 days, and discard any leftovers that have been left out at room temperature for more than 2 hours.

4

Soup Delights

Lentil Soup

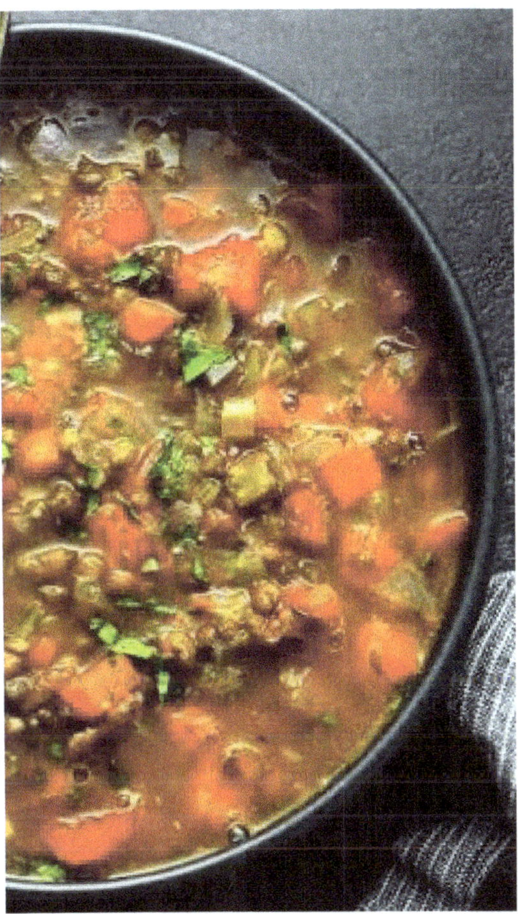

Time of Preparation:

- Approximately 1 hour

Ingredients:

- One cup of washed and drained dried lentils, either brown or green
- 4 cups vegetable broth
- 1 onion, finely chopped
- 2 carrots, diced
- 2 stalks celery, diced
- 3 cloves garlic, minced
- 1 teaspoon ground cumin
- 1 teaspoon ground turmeric
- 1 teaspoon ground coriander
- 1 bay leaf
- Salt and pepper to taste
- 2 tablespoons olive oil

- One can (14.5 ounces) of undrained diced tomatoes
- 2 cups spinach leaves, chopped
- Fresh lemon juice for garnish
- Chopped fresh parsley for garnish

Procedure:

- In a big pot, warm up the olive oil over medium heat. Add chopped onions, carrots, and celery. Simmer the veggies for 5 to 7 minutes, or until they are soft.
- Add minced garlic, cumin, turmeric, coriander, and bay leaf. Cook until aromatic, one or two more minutes.
- Stir in dried lentils, vegetable broth, and diced tomatoes. Bring to a boil, then reduce heat to low. Cover and simmer for about 30-40 minutes, or until lentils are tender.
- Stir in chopped spinach leaves and simmer for an additional 5 minutes until spinach is wilted.

- To taste, add salt and pepper for seasoning. Take off the bay leaf before serving.
- Garnish each serving with a squeeze of fresh lemon juice and chopped parsley.

Tips and Tricks:

- Lentils can be cooked in less time by soaking them overnight.

- Adjust the consistency of the soup by adding more vegetable broth if desired.
- For extra flavor, you can sauté the vegetables in a combination of olive oil and butter.

- Try a variety of herbs and spices to see what suits your palate best.

Nutritional Value per Serving:

- **Calories: 220 kcal**
- **Protein: 13g**
- **Fat: 5g**
- **Carbohydrates: 32g**
- **Fiber: 10g**

Caution and Precautions:

- Be cautious when handling hot liquids to avoid burns.
- Ensure lentils are thoroughly cooked to prevent digestive discomfort.
- Check the expiration date of vegetable broth and canned tomatoes for freshness and safety.

Healthy Additions:

- Add diced potatoes or sweet potatoes for extra heartiness.
- Incorporate chopped kale or Swiss chard for added nutrients.
- Top each serving with a dollop of Greek yogurt for creaminess.

Health Benefits

- Lentils are rich in protein, fiber, and various vitamins and minerals, making them an excellent addition to a healthy diet.
- The combination of vegetables provides a variety of antioxidants and nutrients that support overall health.
- The spices used in the recipe, such as turmeric and cumin, have anti-inflammatory properties and may help boost immunity.

Safety Measures

- Wash hands and all utensils thoroughly before handling ingredients.
- Ensure vegetables are washed properly to remove any dirt or contaminants.
- Use separate cutting boards for vegetables and meats to prevent cross-contamination.

Tomato Basil Soup

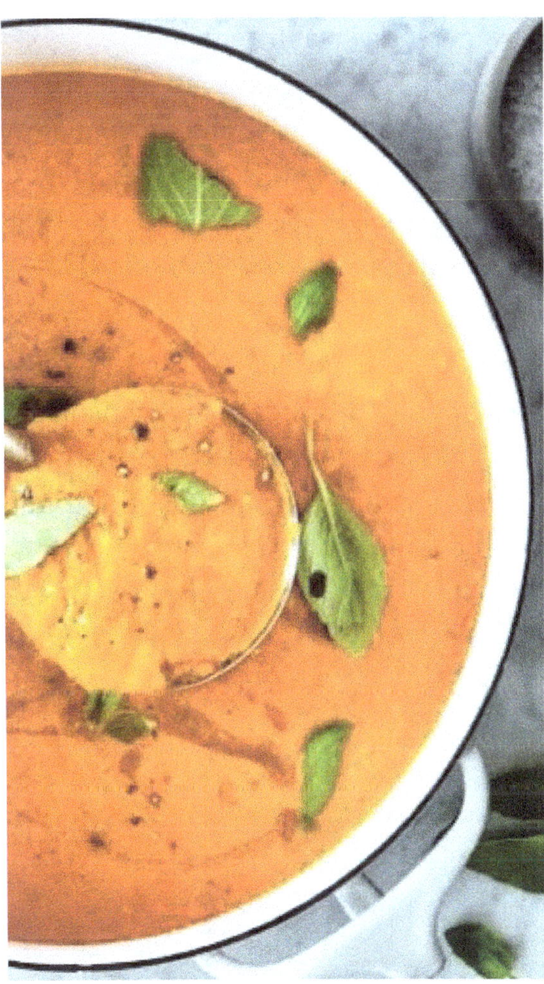

Time of Preparation:

- Approximately 45 minutes

Ingredients:

- 2 tablespoons olive oil
- 1 onion, chopped
- 2 cloves garlic, minced
- 3 cans (28 ounces each) whole tomatoes, undrained
- 1 can (14 ounces) crushed tomatoes
- 4 cups vegetable broth
- 1 cup fresh basil leaves, chopped
- 1 teaspoon dried oregano
- Salt and pepper to taste
- 1/2 cup heavy cream (optional)
- Grated Parmesan cheese for garnish (optional)
- Croutons for serving (optional)

Procedure:

- In a big pot, warm up the olive oil over medium heat. Add chopped onions and simmer for about 5 minutes, or until they become transparent.
- Add the minced garlic and simmer, stirring, for one to two more minutes, or until fragrant.
- Pour in whole tomatoes, crushed tomatoes, and vegetable broth. Bring to a simmer, then reduce heat to low and let it simmer for 20-25 minutes.
- Stir in chopped fresh basil and dried oregano. Season with salt and pepper to taste.

- Blend the soup with an immersion blender until it's smooth. Alternatively, transfer small batches to a blender, blend, and return to the pot.
- If desired, stir in heavy cream for a creamier consistency. Heat through but do not boil.
- Serve hot, garnished with grated Parmesan cheese and croutons if preferred.

Tips and Tricks:

- Use good-quality canned tomatoes for richer flavor.

- Blend the soup and then filter it for a smoother texture.
- Adjust the thickness by adding more broth if needed.
- Fresh basil enhances the flavor, but you can use dried basil if fresh is not available.

Nutritional Value per Serving:

- **Calories: 180 kcal**
- **Protein: 4g**
- **Fat: 10g**
- **Carbohydrates: 20g**
- **Fiber: 5g**

Caution and Precautions:

- Be cautious when blending hot liquids; let the soup cool slightly before blending.

- If salt has been added to canned tomatoes, check and adjust the salt accordingly.

Healthy Addition:

- Boost nutrition by adding a handful of spinach or kale during the simmering process.
- Try incorporating roasted red peppers for a smoky flavor and additional vitamins.

Health Benefits

- Tomatoes are rich in antioxidants like lycopene, which may have potential health benefits.
- Basil contains essential nutrients and may have anti-inflammatory properties.
- The soup is low in calories and can be a good source of hydration.

Safety Measures

- Ensure all utensils and equipment are clean and sanitized.
- Use caution when handling hot soup to avoid burns.
- Store leftovers promptly in the refrigerator.

Butternut Squash Soup

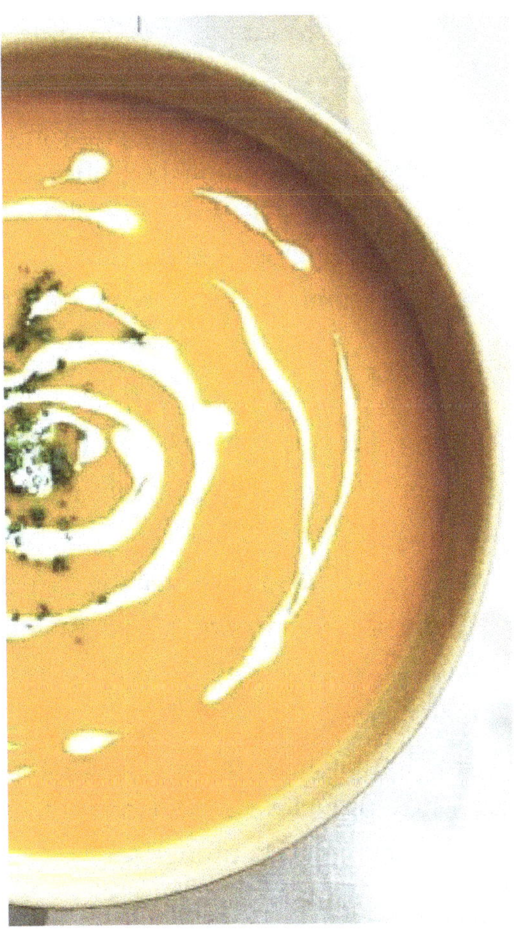

Time of Preparation:

- Approximately 1 hour

Ingredients:

- 1 medium butternut squash (about 3 pounds), peeled, seeded, and cubed
- 2 tablespoons olive oil
- 1 onion, chopped
- 2 carrots, peeled and chopped
- 2 stalks celery, chopped
- 3 cloves garlic, minced
- 4 cups vegetable broth
- 1 teaspoon ground cinnamon
- 1/2 teaspoon ground nutmeg
- Salt and pepper to taste
- 1/2 cup coconut milk (optional)
- Freshly chopped chives or parsley (optional)

Procedure:

- Preheat the oven to 400°F (200°C). Place the cubed butternut squash on a baking sheet, drizzle with olive oil, and season with salt and pepper. Roast in the preheated oven for 25-30 minutes, or until tender and caramelized.

- Olive oil should be heated over medium heat in a big pot.
- Add chopped onions, carrots, and celery. Simmer the vegetables for 5 to 7 minutes, or until they are tender.
- Fry the minced garlic for a further one to two minutes, or until aromatic.
- Add roasted butternut squash cubes to the pot, along with vegetable broth, ground cinnamon, and ground nutmeg. After bringing to a boil, lower the heat and simmer for 15 to 20 minutes.
- Blend the soup with an immersion blender until it's smooth. Alternatively, transfer small batches to a blender, blend, and return to the pot.
- Stir in coconut milk for added creaminess, if desired. Heat through but do not boil.

- Season with additional salt and pepper to taste. If preferred, top with chopped fresh parsley or chives and serve hot.

Tips and Tricks:

- To make peeling and cubing the squash easier, you can briefly microwave it for 2-3 minutes to soften the skin.
- For extra depth of flavor, roast the vegetables (onion, carrot, celery, and garlic) along with the butternut squash.

- You can change the soup's consistency by adding or removing vegetable broth.
- Garnish with a drizzle of balsamic reduction or a sprinkle of toasted pumpkin seeds for added texture and flavor.

Nutritional Value per Serving:

- **Calories: 180 kcal**
- **Protein: 3g**
- **Fat: 10g**
- **Carbohydrates: 22g**
- **Fiber: 5g**

Caution and Precautions:

- Use caution when handling hot trays and equipment during the roasting process.

- To prevent burns, use caution when blending hot liquids.
- Check the seasoning carefully as the amount of salt needed may vary depending on the vegetable broth used.

Healthy Addition:

- Add roasted pears or apples for some sweetness and additional nutrition.
- Top each serving with a dollop of Greek yogurt or sour cream for added creaminess and probiotics.

Health Benefits

- Butternut squash is rich in vitamins A and C, which are essential for immune health and vision.
- The soup is low in calories and contains fiber, making it a satisfying and nutritious option for weight management.
- The combination of vegetables and spices provides antioxidants and anti-inflammatory properties.

Safety Measures

- Wash hands and all utensils thoroughly before handling ingredients.
- Ensure the butternut squash is properly peeled and cubed to prevent accidents while cutting.
- Store leftovers promptly in the refrigerator and consume within a few days.

5

Main Course Dishes

Lemon Herb Grilled Chicken

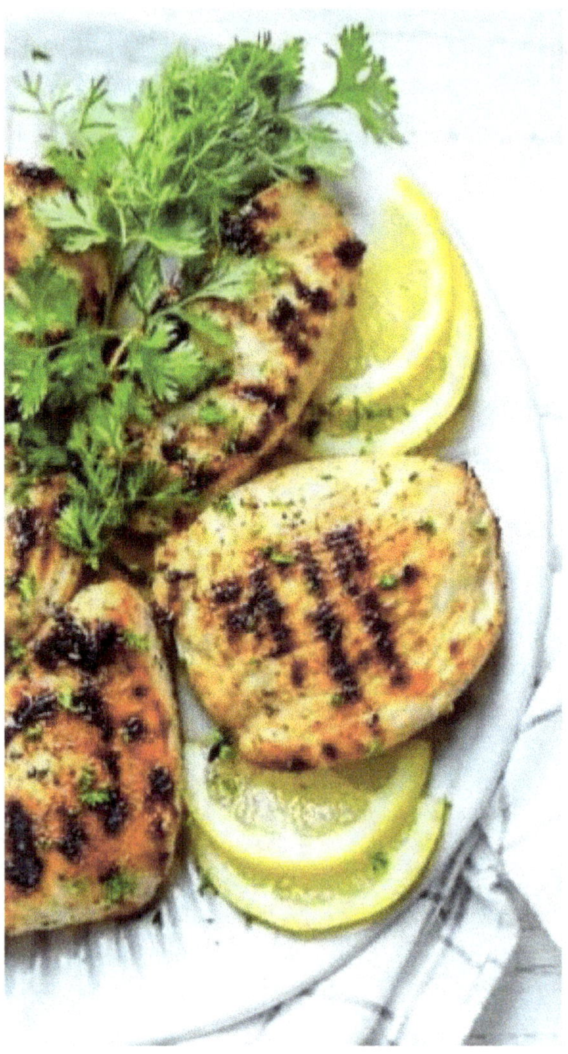

Time of Preparation:

- Preparation Time: 15 minutes
- Marinating Time: 1 hour
- Grilling Time: 10-15 minutes

Ingredients:

- 4 boneless, skinless chicken breasts
- 2 lemons, juiced and zested
- 3 cloves garlic, minced
- 2 tablespoons olive oil
- Two tablespoons of freshly chopped herbs (such oregano, thyme, or rosemary)
- Salt and pepper to taste

Procedure:

- In a small bowl, whisk together lemon juice, lemon zest, minced garlic, olive oil, chopped herbs, salt, and pepper to create the marinade.
- After putting the chicken breasts in a shallow dish or resealable plastic bag, cover them thoroughly with the marinade. For optimal flavor, marinate in the fridge for at least an hour or overnight.
- Preheat the grill to medium-high heat.
- Take the chicken breasts out of the marinade and throw away any leftover marinade.
- Grill the chicken breasts for 5-7 minutes on each side, or until cooked through and no longer pink in the center.
- Remove from the grill and let rest for a few minutes before serving.

Tips and Tricks:

- Pierce the chicken breasts with a fork before marinating to help the flavors penetrate deeper.
- Brush the grill grates with oil before cooking to prevent sticking.
- Avoid overcooking the chicken to maintain its juiciness; use a meat thermometer to ensure it reaches

an internal temperature of 165°F (75°C).

Nutritional Value per Serving:

- **Calories: 250 kcal**
- **Protein: 30g**
- **Fat: 12g**
- **Carbohydrates: 5g**
- **Fiber: 1g**

Caution and Precautions:

- Ensure the chicken is cooked thoroughly to avoid foodborne illness.

- To avoid cross-contamination, use different cutting surfaces and tools for raw and cooked chicken.
- Keep leftovers cold right away to stop bacteria from growing.

Healthy Addition:

- Serve the grilled chicken with a side of steamed vegetables or a fresh salad for a nutritious meal.

Health Benefits

- Lean protein from chicken helps build and repair muscle tissues.
- Lemon juice provides vitamin C, which boosts the immune system and aids in iron absorption.
- Herbs like thyme and rosemary contain antioxidants and may have anti-inflammatory properties.

Safety Measures

- Wash hands and surfaces thoroughly before and after handling raw chicken.

- Refrigerate chicken after marinating it to stop bacterial growth.
- Use fresh lemon juice and herbs for maximum flavor and nutritional benefits.

Baked Salmon with Asparagus

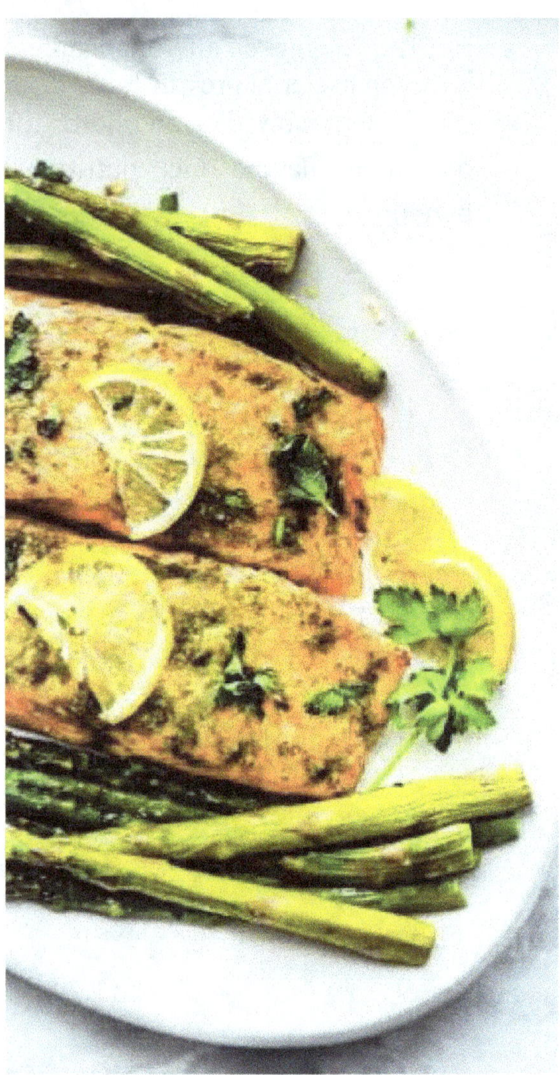

Time of Preparation:

- Preparation Time: 15 minutes
- Baking Time: 15-20 minutes

Ingredients:

- 4 salmon fillets (about 6 ounces each)
- One bunch of asparagus with its rough ends cut
- 2 tablespoons olive oil
- 2 cloves garlic, minced
- 1 lemon, thinly sliced
- Salt and pepper to taste
- Fresh herbs for garnish, such parsley, thyme, or dill

Procedure:

- Preheat the oven to 400°F (200°C).
- Place the salmon fillets and asparagus on a baking sheet lined with parchment paper.
- Drizzle olive oil over the salmon and asparagus. Sprinkle minced garlic evenly over the salmon.
- To taste, add salt and pepper for seasoning. Place lemon slices on top of each salmon fillet.
- Bake in the preheated oven for 15-20 minutes, or until the salmon is cooked through and flakes easily with a fork, and the asparagus is tender but still crisp.
- Garnish with fresh herbs before serving.

Tips and Tricks:

- Choose salmon fillets that are similar in thickness for even cooking.
- If the salmon skin is on, place the fillets skin-side down on the baking sheet.
- To prevent the asparagus from overcooking, you can place them on a separate baking sheet or add them

to the oven halfway through cooking the salmon.

Nutritional Value per Serving:

- **Calories: 300 kcal**
- **Protein: 30g**
- **Fat: 18g**
- **Carbohydrates: 5g**
- **Fiber: 2g**

Caution and Precautions:

- Avoid overcooking the salmon to maintain its moisture and flavor.
- Ensure the salmon reaches an internal temperature of 145°F (63°C) to ensure safe consumption.
- Discard any leftover marinade that has come into contact with raw fish to prevent contamination.

Healthy Addition:

- Serve the baked salmon and asparagus with a side of quinoa or brown rice for a complete and nutritious meal.

Health Benefits

- Salmon is rich in omega-3 fatty acids, which promote heart health and reduce inflammation.
- Asparagus is a good source of fiber, vitamins A, C, and K, and antioxidants that support overall health and immune function.

- Olive oil provides healthy fats and may help reduce the risk of heart disease.

Safety Measures

- Thoroughly wash hands, utensils, and surfaces after handling raw salmon to prevent cross-contamination.
- Use a separate cutting board for preparing raw fish to avoid contamination of other foods.
- Store leftover salmon in an airtight container in the refrigerator and consume within 2-3 days.

Tofu Stir-Fry with Vegetables

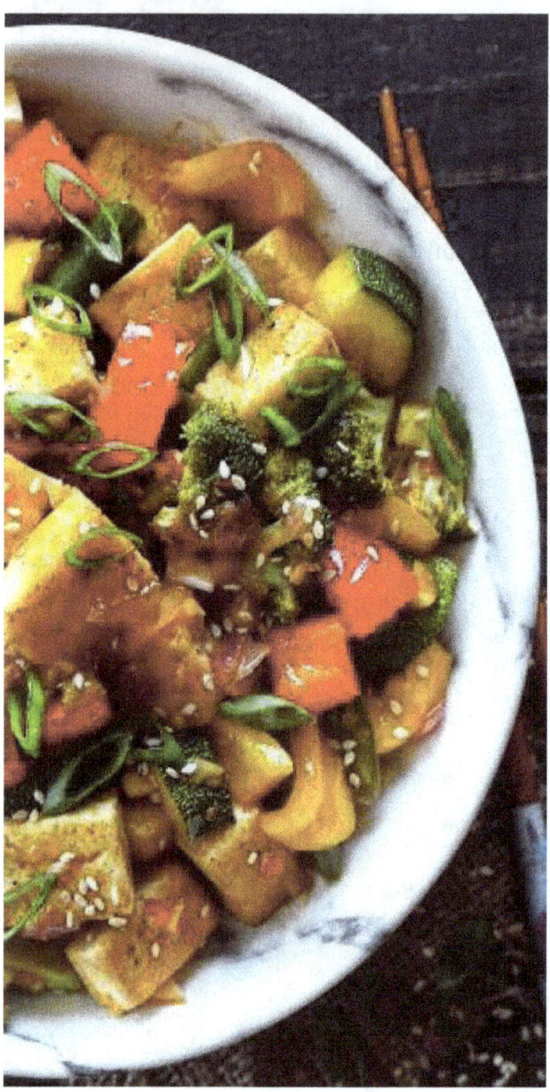

Time of Preparation:

- Preparation Time: 20 minutes
- Cooking Time: 15 minutes

Ingredients:

- 1 block of firm tofu, pressed and cubed
- Two cups of mixed veggies, including snap peas, broccoli, carrots, and bell peppers
- 2 tablespoons soy sauce
- 1 tablespoon sesame oil
- 2 cloves garlic, minced
- 1 tablespoon ginger, minced
- 1 tablespoon cornstarch (optional, for thickening the sauce)
- 2 tablespoons vegetable oil
- Salt and pepper to taste
- Cooked rice or noodles for serving

Procedure:

- In a small bowl, mix soy sauce, sesame oil, minced garlic, minced ginger, and cornstarch (if using). Set aside.

- In a large skillet or wok, heat the vegetable oil over medium-high heat.
- Add cubed tofu to the skillet and cook until golden brown on all sides, about 5-7 minutes. Take out the tofu and place it aside in a skillet.
- In the same skillet, add mixed vegetables and stir-fry for 3-4 minutes, or until they are crisp-tender.
- Return the tofu to the skillet and pour the sauce over the tofu and vegetables. Stir well to coat everything evenly.

- Allow the sauce to slightly thicken by cooking for an additional two to three minutes.
- To taste, add salt and pepper for seasoning.

- Serve hot over cooked rice or noodles.

Tips and Tricks:

- Pressing the tofu before cooking helps remove excess moisture and allows it to absorb more flavors.
- Use a non-stick skillet or wok to prevent the tofu from sticking to the pan.
- For extra flavor, marinate the tofu cubes in soy sauce and sesame oil for 15-20 minutes before cooking.

Nutritional Value per Serving:

- **Calories: 250 kcal**
- **Protein: 15g**
- **Fat: 12g**
- **Carbohydrates: 20g**
- **Fiber: 5g**

Caution and Precautions:

- Be careful when handling hot oil and stirring the ingredients in the skillet to avoid splattering.
- Ensure the tofu is cooked through and has a golden brown crust before adding the vegetables to the skillet.
- Check the labels of store-bought soy sauce and other condiments for added sodium and artificial ingredients.

Healthy Addition:

- Add additional vegetables like mushrooms, zucchini, or spinach for extra nutrients and texture.
- Add some chopped cilantro or green onions as a garnish to give it more taste and freshness.

Health Benefits

- Tofu is a rich source of plant-based protein and contains essential amino acids, making it a nutritious alternative to meat.
- Vegetables provide vitamins, minerals, and dietary fiber essential for overall health and digestion.
- Sesame oil contains antioxidants and healthy fats that may help lower cholesterol levels and reduce inflammation.

Safety Measures

- Use separate cutting boards and utensils for raw tofu and vegetables to prevent cross-contamination.
- Ensure the tofu is cooked to an internal temperature of 165°F (74°C) to kill any harmful bacteria.
- Store leftover tofu stir-fry in an airtight container in the refrigerator for up to 3 days.

Turkey and Vegetable Stir-Fry

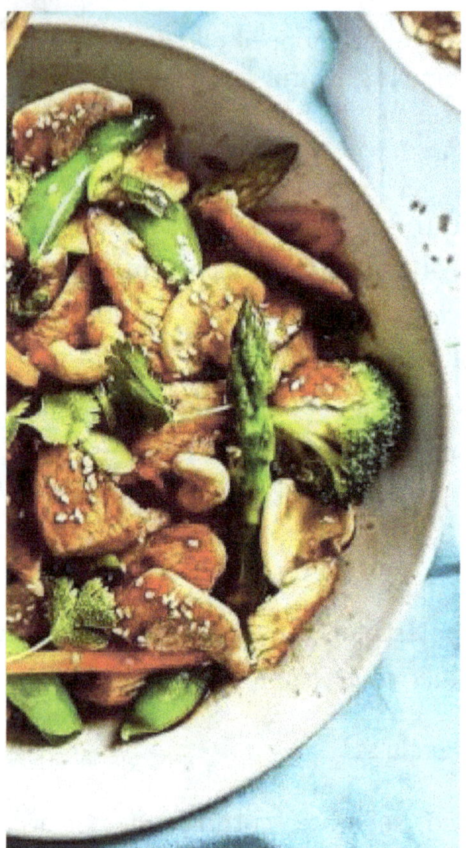

Time of Preparation:

- Preparation Time: 15 minutes
- Cooking Time: 15 minutes

Ingredients:

- 1 lb (450g) ground turkey
- 2 cups mixed vegetables (such as bell peppers, carrots, broccoli, snap peas)
- 2 tablespoons soy sauce
- 1 tablespoon oyster sauce
- 1 tablespoon sesame oil
- 2 cloves garlic, minced
- 1 tablespoon ginger, minced
- 2 tablespoons vegetable oil
- Salt and pepper to taste
- Cooked rice or noodles for serving

Procedure:

- In a large skillet or wok, heat the vegetable oil over medium-high heat.
- Add minced garlic and ginger to the skillet and sauté for 1-2 minutes until fragrant.
- Add ground turkey to the skillet and cook until browned and cooked through, breaking it up with a spatula, about 5-7 minutes.
- Add mixed vegetables to the skillet and stir-fry for 3-4 minutes, or until they are crisp-tender.
- In a small bowl, mix soy sauce, oyster sauce, and sesame oil.
- Pour the sauce over the turkey and vegetables in the skillet. Stir well to coat everything evenly.
- Allow the sauce to slightly thicken by cooking for an additional two to three minutes.
- Season with salt and pepper to taste.
- Serve hot over cooked rice or noodles.

Tips and Tricks:

- For a healthy option, use ground turkey that is lean.
- Stir-fry the vegetables quickly over high heat to retain their crispness and nutrients.

- If the stir-fry appears dry, add a dash of water or chicken broth to help make extra sauce.

Nutritional Value per Serving:

- **Calories: 300 kcal**
- **Protein: 25g**
- **Fat: 15g**
- **Carbohydrates: 15g**
- **Fiber: 3g**

Caution and Precautions:

- Ensure the ground turkey is cooked through and no longer pink in the center to prevent foodborne illness.
- Use separate cutting boards and utensils for raw meat and vegetables to avoid cross-contamination.
- Store leftover turkey and vegetable stir-fry in an airtight container in the refrigerator for up to 3 days.

Healthy Addition:

- Add extra vegetables like mushrooms, snow peas, or spinach for more fiber and nutrients.

- Garnish with sliced green onions or cilantro for added flavor and freshness.

Health Benefits

- Turkey is a lean source of protein and contains essential nutrients like iron, zinc, and B vitamins.
- Vegetables provide vitamins, minerals, and antioxidants that support overall health and immune function.
- Oyster sauce adds depth of flavor without excessive sodium or calories compared to other sauces.

Safety Measures

- Wash hands, utensils, and surfaces thoroughly after handling raw turkey to prevent contamination.
- Cook ground turkey to an internal temperature of 165°F (74°C) to ensure it's safe to eat.
- Use fresh vegetables and herbs for maximum flavor and nutritional benefits.

6

Vegetarian Delicacies

Stuffed Bell Peppers with Quinoa and Black Beans

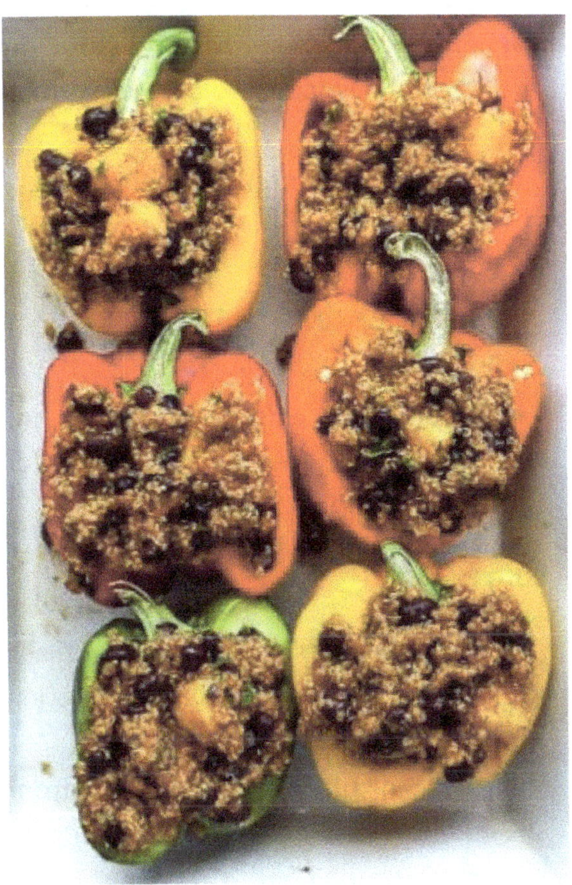

Preparation Time: 45 minutes

- Cooking Time: 30 minutes
- Total Time: 1 hour 15 minutes

Ingredients:

- 4 large bell peppers (any color)
- 1 cup quinoa, rinsed
- One can (15 ounces) of rinsed and drained black beans
- One cup of fresh or frozen corn kernels
- 1 small onion, diced
- 2 cloves garlic, minced
- 1 teaspoon ground cumin
- 1 teaspoon chili powder
- 1/2 teaspoon smoked paprika
- Salt and pepper to taste
- 1 cup of shredded cheese, Monterey Jack, cheddar, or any other type you want
- 1/4 cup fresh cilantro, chopped, for garnish
- Olive oil for cooking
- Optional toppings: avocado slices, sour cream, salsa

Procedure:

- Preheat your oven to 375°F (190°C).
- Prepare the quinoa according to package instructions. Set aside.
- Slice off the bell peppers' tops, then take out the seeds and membranes. Rinse the peppers under cold water and set aside.
- In a large skillet, heat olive oil over medium heat. Add diced onions and cook until translucent, about 3-4 minutes. Sauté the minced garlic for an additional minute.
- Stir in cooked quinoa, black beans, corn, ground cumin, chili powder, smoked paprika, salt, and pepper. Cook for 5-7 minutes until heated through and well combined.
- After taking the skillet off of the burner, add half of the shredded cheese and stir.
- Gently press down to compress the quinoa and black bean mixture into each bell pepper. The filled peppers should be put in a roasting tray.

- Sprinkle the remaining shredded cheese over the stuffed peppers.
- Cover the baking dish with aluminum foil and bake in the preheated oven for 25-30 minutes, until the peppers are tender.
- Remove the foil and bake for an additional 5-10 minutes, until the cheese is melted and bubbly.
- Garnish the stuffed peppers with chopped cilantro and serve hot with optional toppings.

Tips and Tricks:

- Use a variety of bell pepper colors for a visually appealing presentation.
- For extra protein, add cooked ground turkey, chicken, or tofu to the stuffing mixture.
- Customize the seasoning according to your taste preferences by adding herbs like oregano or thyme.
- Make sure to pack the stuffing tightly into the peppers to prevent them from collapsing during baking.

Nutritional Value per Serving:

- **Calories: 350**
- **Total Fat: 10g**
- **Saturated Fat: 5g**
- **Cholesterol: 25mg**
- **Sodium: 450mg**
- **Total Carbohydrates: 50g**
- **Dietary Fiber: 10g**
- **Sugars: 5g**
- **Protein: 15g**

Caution and Precautions:

- Be careful when handling hot peppers and hot baking dishes.
- Ensure the stuffing mixture is thoroughly cooked before stuffing the peppers.
- Allow the stuffed peppers to cool slightly before serving to avoid burns.

Healthy Addition:

- Incorporate diced tomatoes or spinach into the stuffing mixture for added nutrients and flavor.

Health Benefits

- High in fiber from quinoa, black beans, and vegetables, promoting digestive health.
- Rich in plant-based protein from quinoa and black beans, aiding in muscle repair and growth.
- Provides essential vitamins and minerals such as vitamin C, vitamin A, and potassium from bell peppers and other vegetables.
- Low in saturated fat and cholesterol, supporting heart health.
- Suitable for vegetarian and gluten-free diets.

Safety Measures

- Wash hands thoroughly before handling food.
- Ensure all ingredients are fresh and properly rinsed.

- Use separate cutting boards for raw meat (if included) and vegetables to prevent cross-contamination.
- Store leftovers promptly in the refrigerator and consume within 2-3 days.

Eggplant Parmesan

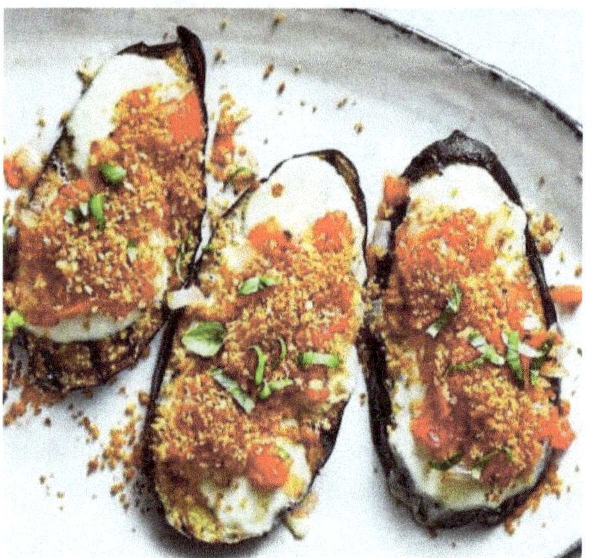

Preparation Time: 30 minutes

- Cooking Time: 45 minutes
- Total Time: 1 hour 15 minutes

Ingredients:

- Half an eggplant each, cut into rounds of half an inch
- 2 cups breadcrumbs (preferably Italian seasoned)
- 1 cup grated Parmesan cheese
- 2 cups marinara sauce
- 2 cups shredded mozzarella cheese
- 2 eggs, beaten
- 1/4 cup chopped fresh basil leaves
- Salt and pepper to taste
- Olive oil for frying
- Optional: fresh parsley for garnish

Procedure:

- Preheat your oven to 375°F (190°C).

- Arrange the eggplant slices on a baking sheet and sprinkle them with salt. To remove extra moisture, let them sit for roughly fifteen minutes.
- Pat the eggplant slices dry with paper towels to remove the excess salt and moisture.
- In a shallow dish, combine breadcrumbs and grated Parmesan cheese.
- Dip each eggplant slice into the beaten eggs, then coat them evenly with the breadcrumb mixture.
- In a large skillet, heat olive oil over medium heat. Fry the breaded eggplant slices in batches until golden brown and crispy on both sides, about 3-4 minutes per side. Transfer the cooked slices to a plate lined with paper towels to drain excess oil.

- Brush the bottom of a baking dish with a thin coating of marinara sauce.
- Place a layer of sauce-covered fried eggplant slices.
- Sprinkle some shredded mozzarella cheese and chopped basil over the eggplant layer.
- Repeat the layers until all the eggplant slices are used, finishing with a layer of marinara sauce and shredded mozzarella cheese on top.

- Bake the baking dish for thirty minutes in a preheated oven covered with aluminum foil.

- After removing the foil, bake the cheese for a further 10 to 15 minutes, or until it is melted and bubbling.
- Garnish with fresh parsley before serving.

Tips and Tricks:

- Use firm, shiny eggplants for the best results.
- Make sure to evenly coat each eggplant slice with breadcrumbs to ensure even frying.
- You can bake the breaded eggplant slices instead of frying them for a healthier alternative.
- To allow the flavors to melt together, let the eggplant parmesan sit for a few minutes before serving.

Nutritional Value per Serving:

- **Calories: 350**
- **Total Fat: 20g**
- **Saturated Fat: 8g**
- **Cholesterol: 70mg**
- **Sodium: 800mg**
- **Total Carbohydrates: 25g**
- **Dietary Fiber: 5g**
- **Sugars: 8g**
- **Protein: 18g**

Caution and Precautions:

- Be careful when frying the eggplant slices to avoid splattering hot oil.
- Watch the eggplant slices closely while frying to prevent them from burning.

- Allow the Eggplant Parmesan to cool slightly before serving to avoid burns.

Healthy Addition:

- Add layers of thinly sliced zucchini or yellow squash along with the eggplant for extra vegetables and nutrients.

Health Benefits

- Eggplants are low in calories and high in fiber, aiding in digestion and promoting weight loss.
- Rich in antioxidants such as vitamins C and E, eggplants help reduce inflammation and lower the risk of chronic diseases.
- Mozzarella cheese provides calcium and protein, essential for bone health and muscle repair.
- Using marinara sauce made with tomatoes provides lycopene, a powerful antioxidant known for its cancer-fighting properties.

Safety Measures

- Wash hands thoroughly before and after handling raw eggplant.
- To avoid cross-contamination, chop raw meat and veggies on different cutting boards.
- Ensure that the eggplant slices are thoroughly cooked to avoid foodborne illness

- Store leftovers promptly in the refrigerator and consume within 2-3 days.

Lentil and Vegetable Curry

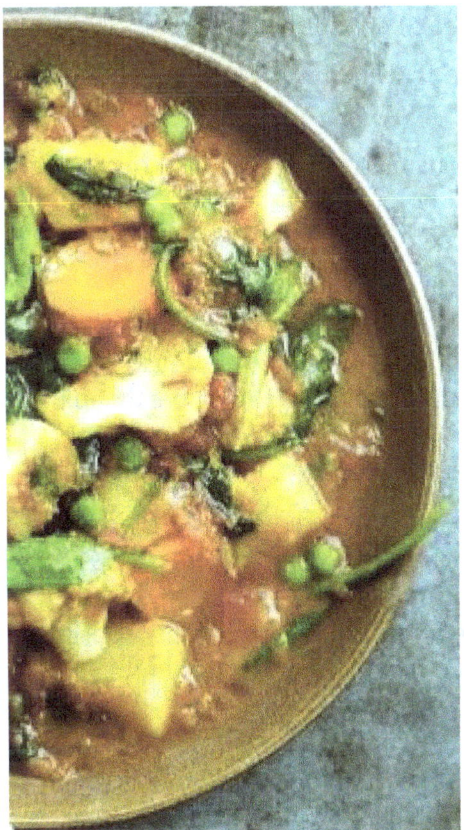

Preparation Time: 15 minutes

- Cooking Time: 45 minutes
- Total Time: 1 hour

Ingredients:

- 1 cup dry lentils (green or brown), rinsed and drained
- 2 tablespoons vegetable oil
- 1 large onion, finely chopped
- 3 cloves garlic, minced
- 1 tablespoon ginger, grated
- 1 red bell pepper, diced
- 1 zucchini, diced
- 1 carrot, diced
- 1 can (14 ounces) diced tomatoes
- 1 can (14 ounces) coconut milk
- 2 tablespoons curry powder
- 1 teaspoon ground cumin
- 1 teaspoon ground coriander
- 1/2 teaspoon turmeric

- Half a teaspoon cayenne, or more, according to taste
- Salt and pepper to taste
- Fresh cilantro, chopped, for garnish
- Cooked rice or naan bread for serving

Procedure:

- In a large pot, combine the rinsed lentils with 4 cups of water. Bring to a boil, then reduce heat, cover, and simmer for 20-25 minutes or until lentils are tender. After removing any extra water, set away.
- In a separate large skillet or pan, heat vegetable oil over medium heat. Add the chopped onions and simmer for 3–4 minutes, or until softened.
- Add minced garlic and grated ginger to the onions, sautéing for an additional minute until fragrant.

- Add curry powder, cayenne pepper, turmeric, ground coriander, and cumin.
- Cook until the spices are well mixed, one to two minutes.
- Add diced bell pepper, zucchini, and carrot to the skillet. Let the vegetables soften by cooking them for five to seven minutes.
- Add the chopped tomatoes and coconut milk, mixing thoroughly. Bring the mixture to a simmer.

- Add the cooked lentils to the vegetable and curry mixture. Season with salt and pepper to taste. Simmer for ten to fifteen more minutes to give the flavors time to mingle.
- Adjust the seasoning if necessary and serve the lentil and vegetable curry over cooked rice or with naan bread.
- Garnish with chopped fresh cilantro before serving.

Tips and Tricks:

- Experiment with different vegetables like spinach, sweet potatoes, or peas for variety.

- You can use full-fat coconut milk for a creamier texture.
- Toast the curry powder and spices in the skillet for a minute before adding vegetables to enhance their flavors.

Nutritional Value per Serving:

- Calories: 350
- Total Fat: 15g
- Saturated Fat: 10g
- Cholesterol: 0mg
- Sodium: 400mg
- Total Carbohydrates: 40g
- Dietary Fiber: 15g
- Sugars: 8g
- Protein: 18g

Caution and Precautions:

- Be cautious when handling hot peppers or spices, especially if using fresh chili peppers.
- Ensure lentils are fully cooked to avoid digestive discomfort.
- If using canned lentils, rinse them thoroughly to reduce sodium content.

Healthy Addition:

- Include a handful of fresh spinach leaves for added vitamins and minerals.

Health Benefits

- Lentils are an excellent source of plant-based protein, fiber, and essential minerals like iron and folate.
- Vegetables provide a range of vitamins and antioxidants, promoting overall health and immune function.
- Coconut milk adds healthy fats and a creamy texture without dairy.
- The combination of spices in curry powder may have anti-inflammatory and digestive benefits.

Safety Measures

- Wash hands thoroughly before handling raw vegetables.
- Ensure lentils are properly cooked to eliminate any potential bacteria.

- Keep leftovers refrigerated and eat them within two to three days.

- To avoid cross-contamination, chop raw meat and veggies on different cutting boards.

7

Healthy Sides

Garlic Roasted Brussels Sprouts

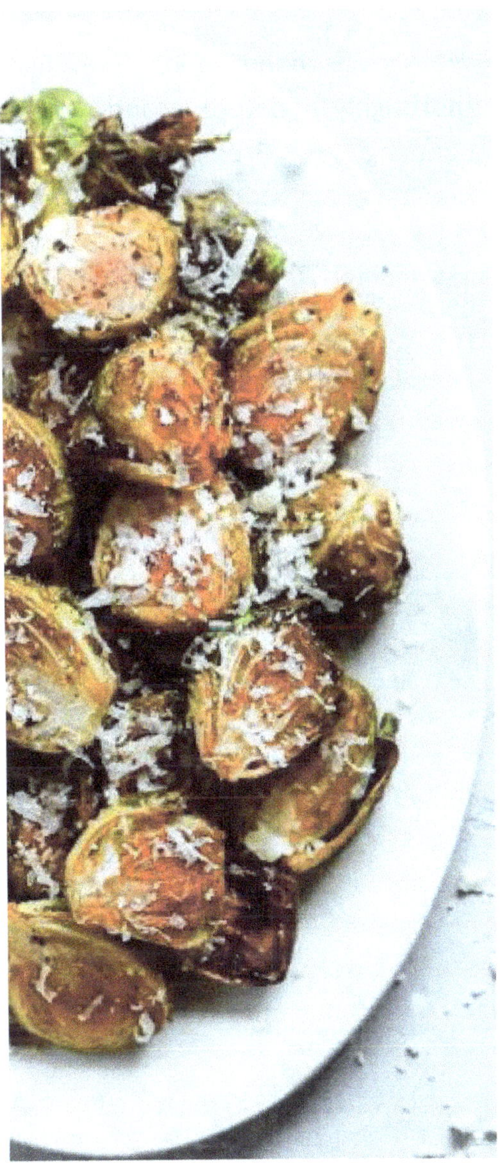

Time of Preparation:

- Preparation Time: 10 minutes
- Cooking Time: 25-30 minutes
- Total Time: 35-40 minutes

Ingredients:

- One pound of halved and trimmed Brussels sprouts
- 3 tablespoons olive oil
- 4 cloves garlic, minced
- Salt and black pepper to taste
- Optional: grated Parmesan cheese for serving

Procedure:

- Preheat your oven to 400°F (200°C).
- In a large mixing bowl, toss Brussels sprouts with olive oil, minced garlic, salt, and pepper until evenly coated.

- Arrange the Brussels sprouts in a single layer on a baking sheet that has been covered with aluminum foil or parchment paper.
- Roast in the preheated oven for 25-30 minutes, or until the Brussels sprouts are tender and caramelized, stirring halfway through to ensure even cooking.
- Once done, remove from the oven and transfer to a serving dish.
- Optionally, sprinkle with grated Parmesan cheese before serving.

Tips and Tricks:

- Ensure the Brussels sprouts are trimmed and halved evenly for uniform cooking.
- Don't overcrowd the baking sheet; give the Brussels sprouts enough space to roast properly.
- Taste and adjust the seasoning to suit your needs.

- Keep an eye on the Brussels sprouts while roasting to prevent burning.

Nutritional Value per Serving (approximate):

- **Calories: 120**
- **Total Fat: 9g**
- **Saturated Fat: 1g**
- **Cholesterol: 0mg**
- **Sodium: 50mg**
- **Total Carbohydrates: 10g**
- **Dietary Fiber: 4g**
- **Sugars: 2g**
- **Protein: 4g**

Caution and Precautions:

- Be careful when handling hot baking sheets and trays.

- To guarantee equal cooking and avoid burning or undercooking, make sure the oven is preheated to the proper temperature.

Healthy Addition:

- Add a squeeze of fresh lemon juice over the roasted Brussels sprouts for a bright and refreshing flavor.

Health Benefits

- Brussels sprouts are rich in vitamins C and K, as well as fiber, and contain antioxidants that may help reduce inflammation and promote heart health.
- Garlic is known for its potential health benefits, including boosting the immune system and reducing the risk of cardiovascular diseases.

Safety Measures

- Wash your hands and all utensils thoroughly before and after handling raw Brussels sprouts to prevent cross-contamination.

- To eradicate any potentially hazardous bacteria, make sure the Brussels sprouts are roasted to an internal temperature of 165°F (74°C).

Steamed Broccoli with Lemon

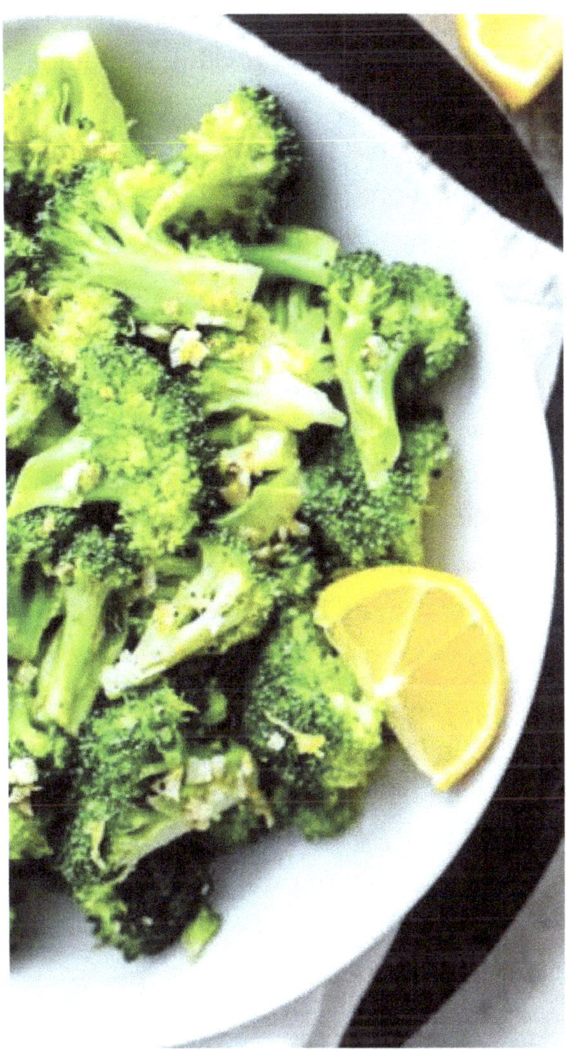

Time of Preparation:

- Preparation Time: 5 minutes
- Cooking Time: 5-7 minutes
- Total Time: 10-12 minutes

Ingredients:

- 1 pound fresh broccoli, cut into florets
- 1 tablespoon olive oil
- 2 tablespoons freshly squeezed lemon juice
- Salt and black pepper to taste
- Lemon zest for garnish (optional)

Procedure:

- Prepare a steamer basket by filling a pot with 1-2 inches of water and bringing it to a boil over medium heat.
- Place the broccoli florets in the steamer basket and cover the pot with a lid.
- Steam the broccoli for 5-7 minutes, or until tender but still crisp.
- While the broccoli is steaming, in a small bowl, whisk together the olive oil and lemon juice.
- Once the broccoli is steamed, transfer it to a serving dish and drizzle the lemon and olive oil mixture over the top.
- To taste, add salt and black pepper for seasoning.
- Garnish with lemon zest if desired.
- Serve hot and enjoy!

Tips and Tricks:

- Don't overcook the broccoli; it should be vibrant green and still slightly crisp to maintain its nutrients and texture.
- If you don't have a steamer basket, you can also steam the broccoli in a microwave-safe dish with a little

water, covered with plastic wrap or a microwave-safe lid.

- To enhance the flavor, you can add minced garlic or red pepper flakes to the olive oil and lemon juice mixture before drizzling it over the broccoli.

Nutritional Value per Serving (approximate):

- **Calories: 60**
- **Total Fat: 4g**
- **Saturated Fat: 0.5g**
- **Cholesterol: 0mg**
- **Sodium: 40mg**
- **Total Carbohydrates: 6g**
- **Dietary Fiber: 3g**
- **Sugars: 2g**
- **Protein: 3g**

Caution and Precautions:

- Use caution when handling hot steam and boiling water to prevent burns.
- Make sure the broccoli is thoroughly washed before steaming to remove any dirt or debris.
- Healthy Addition:
- Sprinkle toasted sesame seeds or chopped almonds over the steamed broccoli for added crunch and nutty flavor.

Health Benefits

- Broccoli is a nutrient-rich vegetable packed with vitamins C, K, and A, as well as fiber and antioxidants, which may help support a healthy immune system and reduce the risk of chronic diseases.
- Lemon juice adds a refreshing citrus flavor and provides additional vitamin C, which is essential for collagen synthesis and immune function.

Safety Measures

- Always use clean utensils and cutting boards when preparing fresh vegetables to prevent contamination.
- Make sure the broccoli is cooked to a safe temperature and avoid consuming it if it has a strong odor or shows signs of spoilage.

Quinoa Pilaf

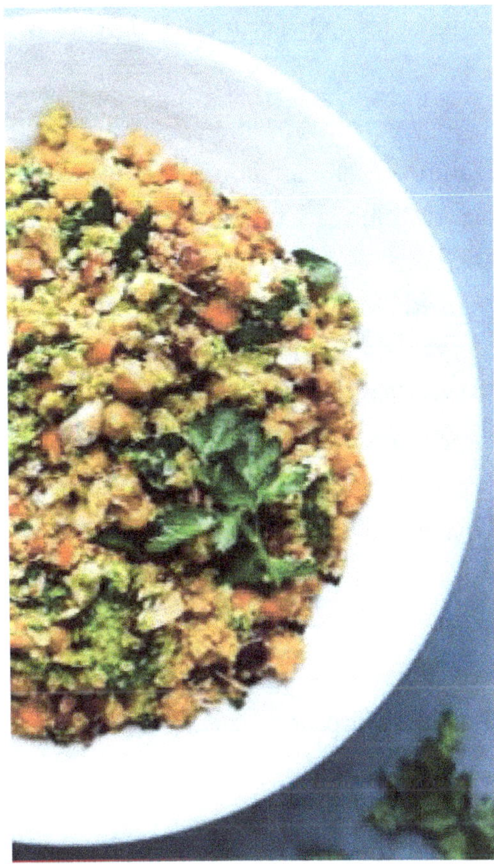

Time of Preparation:

- Preparation Time: 10 minutes
- Cooking Time: 25-30 minutes
- Total Time: 35-40 minutes

Ingredients:

- 1 cup quinoa, rinsed
- 2 cups vegetable broth or water
- 1 tablespoon olive oil
- 1 small onion, finely chopped
- 2 cloves garlic, minced
- 1 carrot, diced
- 1 bell pepper, diced
- 1/2 cup peas (fresh or frozen)
- Salt and pepper to taste
- 1/4 cup chopped fresh parsley or cilantro (optional, for garnish)

Procedure:

- Quinoa should be combined with water or vegetable broth in a medium-sized saucepan. Bring to a boil, then reduce the heat to low, cover, and simmer for 15-20 minutes, or until the quinoa is cooked and the liquid is absorbed. Take it off the heat and leave it covered for five minutes.
- While the quinoa is cooking, heat the olive oil in a large skillet over medium heat. Add the chopped onion and cook until translucent, about 3-4 minutes.
- Once aromatic, add the minced garlic and simmer for an additional minute.
- Stir in the diced carrot, bell pepper, and peas. Cook the vegetables for five to seven minutes, or until they are crisp-tender.
- Once the quinoa is done, fluff it with a fork and transfer it to the skillet with the cooked vegetables. Stir to combine.

- To taste, add salt and pepper for seasoning.
- Before serving, garnish with chopped cilantro or fresh parsley, if preferred.

Tips and Tricks:

- Before cooking, give the quinoa a thorough rinse to get rid of any bitter flavor.
- For extra taste, use vegetable broth in place of water.

- You can alter the vegetables to suit your tastes or what you have on hand.
- Before adding the liquid, you can toast the quinoa in the skillet for more flavor.

Nutritional Value per Serving (approximate):

- **Calories: 220**
- **Total Fat: 6g**
- **Saturated Fat: 1g**
- **Cholesterol: 0mg**
- **Sodium: 400mg**
- **Total Carbohydrates: 35g**
- **Dietary Fiber: 5g**
- **Sugars: 4g**
- **Protein: 8g**

Caution and Precautions:

- Be careful when handling hot pans and utensils to prevent burns.
- Make sure the quinoa is cooked thoroughly to avoid any risk of foodborne illness.
- Healthy Addition:

- Add a handful of toasted nuts or seeds, such as almonds or pumpkin seeds, for extra crunch and protein.

Health Benefits

- Quinoa is a complete protein, containing all nine essential amino acids, making it an excellent plant-based source of protein for vegetarians and vegans.
- This dish is rich in fiber, vitamins, and minerals from the vegetables, contributing to digestive health and overall well-being.

Safety Measures

- Wash all vegetables thoroughly before chopping to remove any dirt or pesticides.

- Any leftovers should be eaten within three to four days after being refrigerated in an airtight container.

8

Guilt-Free Desserts

Mixed Berry Chia Seed Pudding

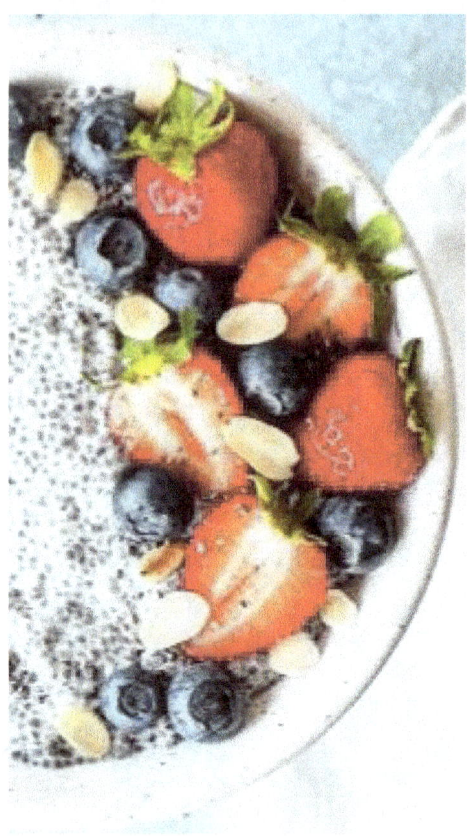

Time of Preparation:

- Approximately 10 minutes (plus chilling time).

Ingredients:

- 1/4 cup chia seeds

- One cup of mixed berries, including raspberries, blueberries, and strawberries
- 1 1/2 cups unsweetened almond milk (or any milk of your choice)
- 1 tablespoon honey or maple syrup (optional, for sweetness)
- 1 teaspoon vanilla extract
- Fresh mint leaves for garnish (optional)

Procedure:

- In a mixing bowl, combine chia seeds, almond milk, honey (if using), and vanilla extract. Stir well to combine.
- Let the mixture sit for about 5 minutes, then stir again to break up any clumps of chia seeds.
- Cover the bowl and refrigerate for at least 2 hours or overnight, allowing the chia seeds to absorb the liquid and thicken into a pudding-like consistency.
- Before serving, wash and prepare the mixed berries. If using strawberries, remove the stems and slice them.
- Divide the chia seed pudding into serving glasses or bowls.
- Top each serving with a generous amount of mixed berries.
- If desired, garnish with fresh mint leaves.
- Serve chilled and enjoy!

Tips and Tricks:

- For a smoother pudding texture, blend the almond milk and mixed berries before adding the chia seeds.
- Adjust sweetness according to your preference by adding more or less honey or maple syrup.

- Experiment with different types of milk like coconut milk or oat milk for variety.
- Make sure to stir the chia seed mixture well, especially after the first few minutes, to prevent clumping.
- Allow the pudding to chill for at least 2 hours, or preferably overnight, for the best consistency.

Nutritional Value per Serving:

- **Calories: 180 kcal**
- **Total Fat: 8g**
- **Saturated Fat: 1g**
- **Cholesterol: 0mg**
- **Sodium: 100mg**
- **Total Carbohydrates: 24g**
- **Dietary Fiber: 10g**
- **Sugars: 10g**
- **Protein: 5g**

Caution and Precautions:

- If you have any allergies to chia seeds or berries, avoid consuming this recipe.
- Always check the expiration dates of your ingredients, especially the almond milk, to ensure freshness and safety.

- Any leftovers should be eaten within two to three days after being refrigerated in an airtight container.

Healthy Addition:

- Add a tablespoon of unsweetened shredded coconut or chopped nuts for added texture and flavor.

Health Benefits

- Chia seeds are packed with omega-3 fatty acids, fiber, protein, and various nutrients, promoting heart health, digestion, and weight management.
- Mixed berries are rich in antioxidants, vitamins, and minerals, supporting immune function, skin health, and reducing inflammation.

Safety Measures

- Wash your hands thoroughly before handling food ingredients.
- Use clean utensils and kitchen equipment to prevent contamination.
- Store perishable ingredients like berries in the refrigerator to maintain freshness and reduce the risk of spoilage.
- Practice good food safety habits by storing leftovers promptly and at the correct temperature.

Dark Chocolate Avocado Mousse

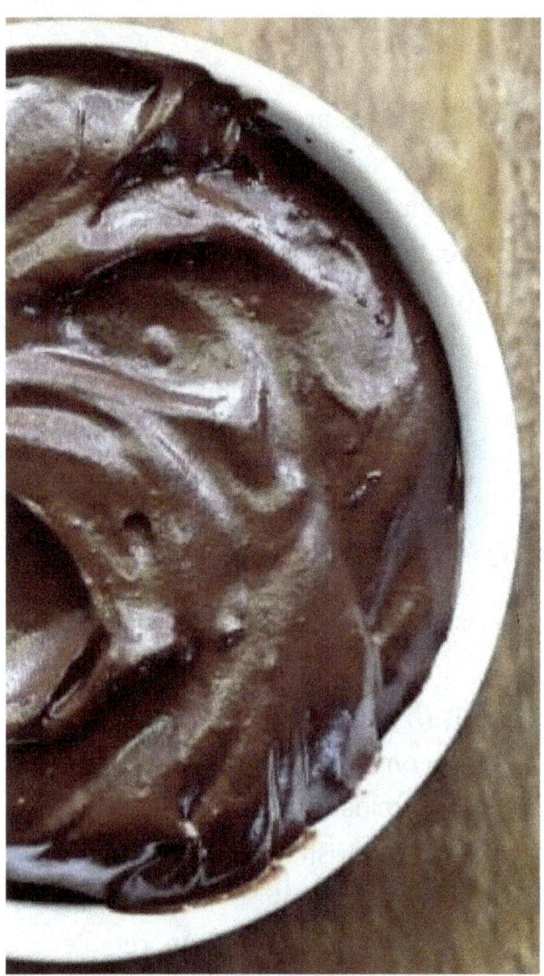

Time of Preparation:

- Approximately 15 minutes.

Ingredients:

- 2 ripe avocados
- 1/4 cup unsweetened cocoa powder
- 1/4 cup maple syrup or honey
- 1 teaspoon vanilla extract
- Pinch of salt
- 1/4 cup almond milk (or any other type of milk)
- Dark chocolate shavings or cocoa nibs for garnish (optional)

Procedure:

- Remove the pits from the avocados, cut them in half, and scoop out the meat into a food processor or blender.
- Add cocoa powder, maple syrup or honey, vanilla extract, salt, and almond milk to the blender.

- Using a food processor or blender to scrape down the sides as necessary, mix the ingredients until they are smooth and creamy.
- Taste the mousse and adjust the sweetness or cocoa flavor to your liking by adding more maple syrup/honey or cocoa powder if necessary.
- Once the mixture is smooth and well combined, transfer it to serving bowls or glasses.

- To prevent oxidation, cover the mousse with plastic wrap, making sure it reaches the surface, and chill it in the refrigerator for at least half an hour.
- Before serving, garnish with dark chocolate shavings or cocoa nibs if desired.
- Enjoy your indulgent and healthy dark chocolate avocado mousse!

Tips and Tricks:

- Use ripe avocados for the creamiest texture and best flavor.
- Adjust the sweetness according to your taste preferences by adding more or less maple syrup/honey.
- For a thicker mousse, use less almond milk, and for a thinner consistency, add more almond milk.
- Make sure to blend the ingredients until completely smooth to avoid any avocado chunks in the mousse.
- Chill the mousse in the refrigerator for at least 30 minutes before serving to allow the flavors to meld together.

Nutritional Value per Serving:

- **Calories: 200 kcal**
- **Total Fat: 15g**
- **Saturated Fat: 2g**
- **Cholesterol: 0mg**
- **Sodium: 10mg**
- **Total Carbohydrates: 20g**
- **Dietary Fiber: 7g**
- **Sugars: 10g**
- **Protein: 3g**

Caution and Precautions:

- Make sure the avocados are ripe and free from any signs of spoilage before using them in the recipe.
- If you have a known allergy to avocados or cocoa, avoid consuming this recipe.

- Any leftovers should be eaten within two to three days after being refrigerated in an airtight container.

Healthy Addition:

- Top the mousse with fresh berries or sliced bananas for added freshness and nutrition.

Health Benefits

- Avocados are rich in healthy fats, fiber, and vitamins, promoting heart health, digestion, and skin health.
- Dark chocolate is high in antioxidants, flavonoids, and minerals, supporting brain function, mood, and reducing inflammation.

Safety Measures

- Wash your hands thoroughly before handling food ingredients.
- Use clean utensils and kitchen equipment to prevent contamination.
- Store perishable ingredients like avocados in the refrigerator to maintain freshness and reduce the risk of spoilage.
- Ensure that the blender or food processor is clean and dry before blending the ingredients.

Banana Oatmeal Cookies

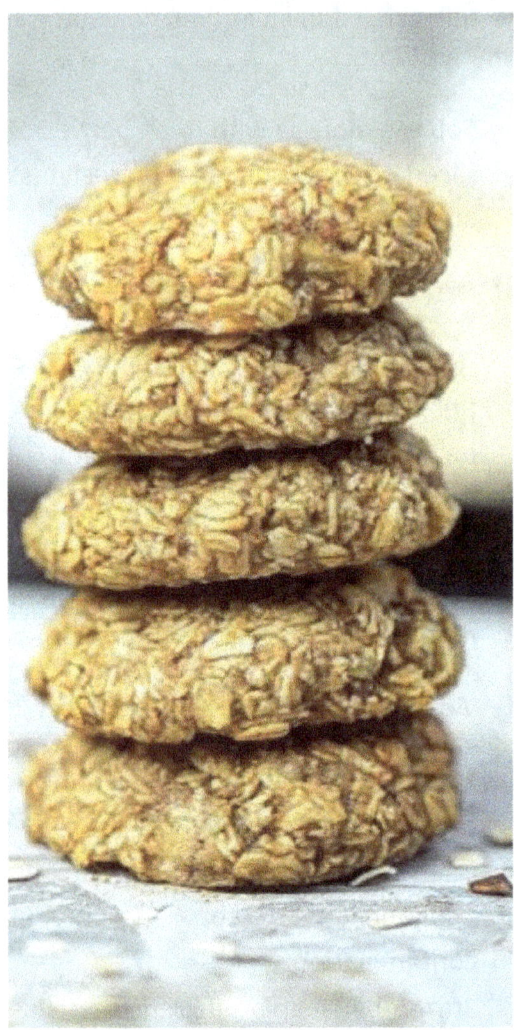

Time of Preparation:

- Approximately 20 minutes.

Ingredients:

- 2 ripe bananas, mashed
- 1 1/2 cups rolled oats
- 1/2 cup unsweetened applesauce
- 1/4 cup almond butter or peanut butter
- 1/4 cup raisins or chocolate chips (optional)
- 1 teaspoon vanilla extract
- 1 teaspoon cinnamon
- Pinch of salt

Procedure:

- Adjust the oven temperature to 350°F (175°C) and place parchment paper on a baking pan.
- In a large mixing bowl, combine mashed bananas, rolled oats, applesauce, almond butter or peanut butter, vanilla extract, cinnamon, and a pinch of salt. Stir thoroughly to include all of the ingredients.
- If using, fold in raisins or chocolate chips into the cookie dough mixture.
- Using a spoon or cookie scoop, drop dollops of the cookie dough onto the prepared baking sheet, spacing them evenly apart.
- Flatten each cookie slightly with the back of a spoon or your fingers, as they will not spread much during baking.
- Bake in the preheated oven for 12-15 minutes, or until the cookies are golden brown around the edges.
- Once done, remove from the oven and let the cookies cool on the baking sheet for a few minutes before transferring them to a wire rack to cool completely.
- Enjoy your healthy and delicious banana oatmeal cookies!

Tips and Tricks:

- To get the maximum flavor and sweetness, use ripe bananas with brown patches.
- Customize your cookies by adding your favorite mix-ins such as chopped nuts, dried fruits, or shredded coconut.
- If the cookie dough seems too wet, add more oats. If it's too dry, add a splash of almond milk or water to adjust the consistency.
- For extra flavor, toast the rolled oats in the oven for a few minutes before mixing them into the dough.
- Make sure to flatten the cookies slightly before baking to ensure even cooking.

Nutritional Value per Serving:

- **Calories: 100 kcal**
- **Total Fat: 3g**
- **Saturated Fat: 0.5g**
- **Cholesterol: 0mg**
- **Sodium: 20mg**
- **Total Carbohydrates: 17g**
- **Dietary Fiber: 2g**
- **Sugars: 6g**
- **Protein: 2g**

Caution and Precautions:

- If you have a known allergy to any of the ingredients, especially nuts or chocolate, avoid consuming this recipe.

- Any leftovers can be frozen for longer storage or kept at room temperature for up to 3–4 days in an airtight container.
- Be mindful of portion sizes as these cookies are still a treat and can contribute to excess calorie intake if consumed in large quantities.

Healthy Addition:

- Add a tablespoon of ground flaxseed or chia seeds for added fiber and omega-3 fatty acids.

Health Benefits

- Rich in potassium, vitamins, and fiber, bananas promote healthy digestion, heart health, and muscular performance.
- Oats are rich in fiber, antioxidants, and complex carbohydrates, promoting satiety, blood sugar control, and digestive health.

Safety Measures

- Wash your hands thoroughly before handling food ingredients.
- Use clean utensils and kitchen equipment to prevent contamination.
- Store perishable ingredients like bananas and applesauce in the refrigerator to maintain freshness.
- Ensure that the baking sheet is lined with parchment paper to prevent sticking and facilitate easy cleanup.

9

Beverages

Refreshing Cucumber Mint Water

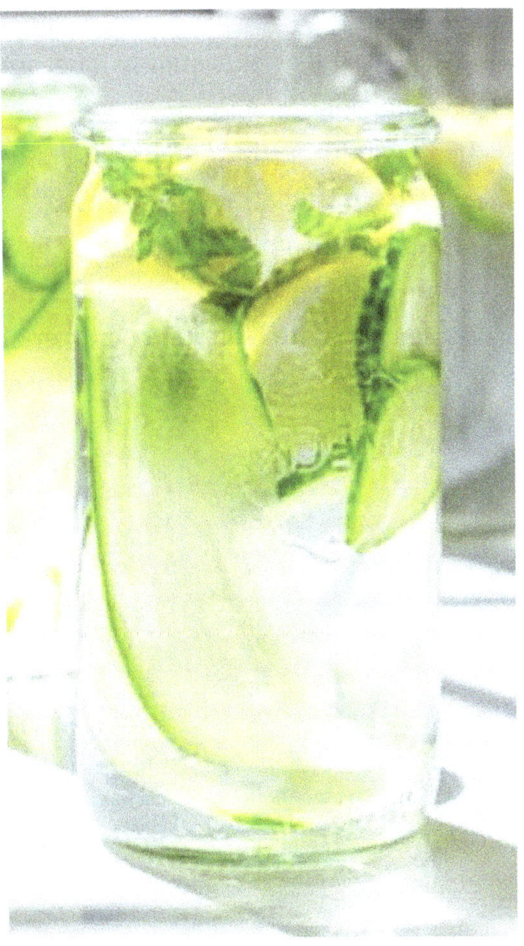

Time of Preparation:

- Preparation Time: 10 minutes
- Infusion Time: 1-2 hours
- Total Time: 1 hour 10 minutes to 2 hours 10 minutes

Ingredients:

- 1 medium cucumber, thinly sliced
- 1/4 cup fresh mint leaves, washed
- 8 cups of filtered water
- Ice cubes (optional)
- Lemon slices (optional, for garnish)

Procedure:

- Wash the cucumber thoroughly under running water and slice it thinly.
- Wash the mint leaves and gently crush them to release their aroma.
- In a large pitcher, add the sliced cucumber and mint leaves.
- After adding the filtered water, gently whisk the ingredients together.
- Cover the pitcher and let it infuse in the refrigerator for 1-2 hours for the flavors to meld.
- Once infused, serve the cucumber mint water over ice cubes, garnished with lemon slices if desired.

Tips and Tricks:

- For a stronger flavor, you can lightly muddle the cucumber slices and mint leaves before adding water.
- For optimal flavor and nutritional content, choose organic and freshly-picked foods.
- Adjust the amount of cucumber and mint according to your preference for flavor intensity.
- Prepare the cucumber mint water fresh for optimal taste and freshness.

Nutritional Value per Serving (1 cup):

- **Calories: 0**
- **Total Fat: 0g**

- **Cholesterol: 0mg**
- **Sodium: 0mg**
- **Total Carbohydrates: 0g**
- **Dietary Fiber: 0g**
- **Sugars: 0g**
- **Protein: 0g**

Caution and Precautions:

- Ensure that the cucumber and mint leaves are thoroughly washed to remove any dirt or contaminants.
- If using store-bought cucumbers, consider peeling them to remove any wax coating.
- Discard the water if it has been left at room temperature for more than 2 hours to prevent bacterial growth.

Healthy Addition:

- You can add a few slices of fresh ginger for an extra kick of flavor and potential health benefits.
- Health Benefits of this Recipe:
- Hydration: Cucumber mint water helps keep you hydrated, which is essential for overall health and well-being.
- Antioxidants: Mint leaves contain antioxidants that can help protect cells from damage caused by free radicals.
- Digestive Health: Cucumber is rich in fiber, which aids digestion and promotes bowel regularity.
- Low in Calories: This refreshing drink is a low-calorie alternative to sugary beverages, making it a healthier choice for hydration.

Safety Measures

- Wash hands thoroughly before handling ingredients.
- Use clean utensils and containers to avoid contamination.
- Store the cucumber mint water in a clean, covered pitcher in the refrigerator to prevent bacterial growth.

Homemade Ginger Turmeric Tea

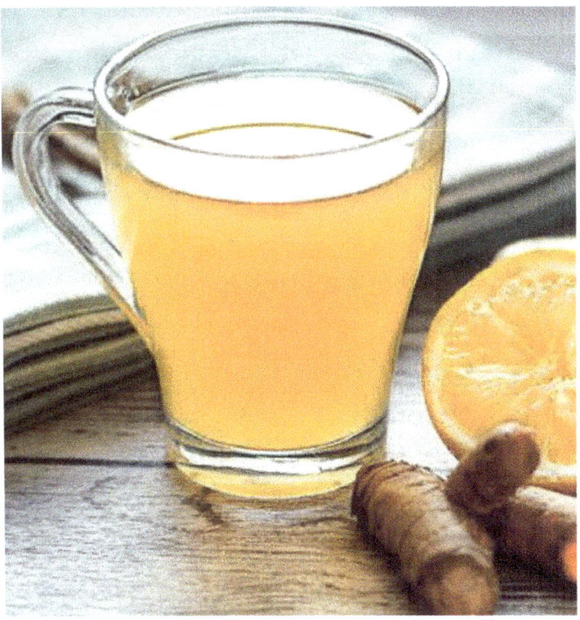

Time of Preparation:

- Preparation Time: 5 minutes
- Cooking Time: 10 minutes
- Total Time: 15 minutes

Ingredients:

- 2 cups of water

- One tablespoon of freshly grated and peeled ginger
- 1 teaspoon fresh turmeric root, peeled and grated (or 1/2 teaspoon ground turmeric)
- 1-2 teaspoons honey or maple syrup (optional, for sweetness)
- 1/2 lemon, juiced (optional, for flavor)

- A pinch of black pepper (optional; improves absorption of turmeric)

- 1 cinnamon stick (optional, for added flavor)

Procedure:

- In a small saucepan, bring the water to a boil over medium heat.

- To the boiling water, add the turmeric and grated ginger.
- Reduce the heat to low and let the mixture simmer for about 5-10 minutes, allowing the flavors to infuse.
- If using, add honey or maple syrup, lemon juice, black pepper, and cinnamon stick to the tea. Stir well to combine.
- Remove the saucepan from heat and strain the tea into cups using a fine mesh strainer.
- Serve the ginger turmeric tea hot and enjoy!

Tips and Tricks:

- Adjust the amount of ginger and turmeric according to your taste preferences.
- Use fresh ginger and turmeric for the best flavor and nutritional benefits.
- If you prefer a smoother texture, you can blend the ginger and turmeric with water before simmering.
- Experiment with different variations by adding ingredients like orange

peel, cardamom pods, or cloves for unique flavors.

Nutritional Value per Serving:

- **Calories: 10**
- **Total Fat: 0g**
- **Cholesterol: 0mg**
- **Sodium: 0mg**
- **Total Carbohydrates: 3g**
- **Dietary Fiber: 0g**
- **Sugars: 2g**
- **Protein: 0g**

Caution and Precautions:

- Be cautious when handling fresh turmeric as it can stain clothes and countertops.
- Consult with a healthcare professional before consuming turmeric if you are pregnant, nursing, or taking medications, as it may interact with certain drugs.
- Turmeric may cause gastrointestinal discomfort in some individuals if consumed in large quantities.

Healthy Addition:

- You can add a slice of fresh ginger or turmeric to each cup as a garnish for extra flavor and visual appeal.

Health Benefits

- Anti-inflammatory Properties: Both ginger and turmeric have potent anti-inflammatory properties that can help reduce inflammation in the body.
- Immune Boosting: Ginger and turmeric are rich in antioxidants and vitamins that support immune function and help the body fight off infections.
- Digestive Aid: Ginger has long been used to aid digestion and alleviate symptoms of indigestion and bloating.
- Antioxidant-rich: Turmeric contains curcumin, a powerful antioxidant that helps neutralize free radicals and protect cells from damage.

Safety Measures

- Wash hands and utensils thoroughly before handling ingredients.
- Use a clean saucepan and strainer to prevent contamination.
- Store any leftover tea in a sealed container in the refrigerator for up to 2 days.

Berry Blast Smoothie

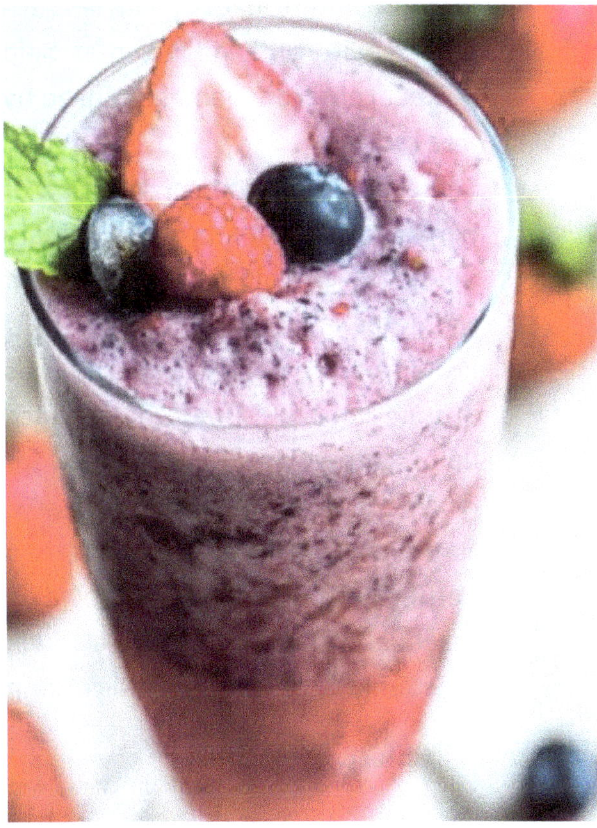

Time of Preparation:

- Preparation Time: 5 minutes
- Total Time: 5 minutes

Ingredients:

- One cup of mixed berries, including raspberries, blueberries, and strawberries
- 1 ripe banana, peeled and sliced
- 1/2 cup plain Greek yogurt
- Half a cup almond milk, or any other type of milk you prefer
- 1 tablespoon honey or maple syrup (optional, for sweetness)
- Half a teaspoon of optional vanilla essence (for flavor)

Procedure:

- Add the mixed berries, sliced banana, Greek yogurt, almond milk, honey or maple syrup, and vanilla extract to a blender.
- If necessary, scrape down the edges of the mixer as you blend on high speed until the mixture is smooth and creamy.
- Taste the smoothie and adjust the sweetness or thickness by adding more honey, milk, or yogurt as desired.
- Once the desired consistency is reached, pour the berry blast smoothie into glasses and serve immediately.

Tips and Tricks:

- Use frozen berries for a thicker and colder smoothie without the need for ice cubes.
- For added protein, you can include a scoop of protein powder or a handful of spinach leaves.
- Customize the smoothie by adding ingredients like chia seeds, flaxseeds, or nut butter for extra nutrition and texture.
- To make the smoothie creamier, freeze the banana slices beforehand.

Nutritional Value per Serving:

- Calories: 150

- **Total Fat: 2g**
- **Cholesterol: 5mg**
- **Sodium: 40mg**
- **Total Carbohydrates: 30g**
- **Dietary Fiber: 4g**
- **Sugars: 20g**
- **Protein: 7g**

Caution and Precautions:

- Be cautious when blending hot liquids as the pressure can cause the lid to pop off. Gradually raise the speed of blending after starting on low.
- If using frozen berries, be mindful of brain freeze if consuming the smoothie too quickly.
- Check for any allergies to berries, dairy, or other ingredients before consuming.

Healthy Addition:

- Add a handful of spinach or kale for added vitamins and minerals without altering the flavor significantly.

Health Benefits

- Rich in Antioxidants: Berries are packed with antioxidants that help protect cells from damage caused by free radicals.
- Source of Fiber: The combination of berries and banana provides dietary fiber, which aids digestion and promotes satiety.
- Protein-Rich: Greek yogurt adds protein to the smoothie, which helps keep you full and satisfied for longer.
- Nutrient Dense: This smoothie is a nutrient powerhouse, providing essential vitamins and minerals such as vitamin C, potassium, and calcium.

Safety Measures

- Wash hands and fruits thoroughly before preparation.
- Use clean utensils and blender to prevent contamination.
- Store any leftover smoothie in a sealed container in the refrigerator for up to 24 hours.

10

Meal Plan

14-Day Healthy Meal Plan

Day 1:

- Breakfast: Green Smoothie Bowl
- Lunch: Lentil Soup
- Dinner: Steamed broccoli and Grilled Chicken with Lemon Herbs

Day 2:

- Breakfast: Avocado Toast with Poached Egg
- Lunch: Greek Yogurt Veggie Dip with Crudites
- Dinner: Baked Salmon with Asparagus

Day 3:

- Breakfast: Quinoa Breakfast Bowl
- Lunch: Kale and Quinoa Salad
- Dinner: Tofu Stir-Fry with Vegetables

Day 4:

- Breakfast: Mixed Berry Chia Seed Pudding
- Lunch: Mediterranean Chickpea Salad
- Dinner: Turkey and Vegetable Stir-Fry

Day 5:

- Breakfast: Berry Blast Smoothie
- Lunch: Lentil and Vegetable Curry
- Dinner: Black beans and Quinoa Stuffed Bell Peppers
- **Day 6:**

- Breakfast: Dark Chocolate Avocado Mousse
- Lunch: Hummus with Crudites
- Dinner: Eggplant Parmesan

Day 7:

- Breakfast: Banana Oatmeal Cookies
- Lunch: Tomato Basil Soup
- Dinner: Garlic Roasted Brussels Sprouts with Quinoa Pilaf

Day 8:

- Breakfast: Quinoa Breakfast Bowl
- Lunch: Spinach and Strawberry Salad
- Dinner: Baked Salmon with Asparagus

Day 9:

- Breakfast: Green Smoothie Bowl
- Lunch: Lentil Soup
- Dinner: Steamed broccoli and Grilled Chicken with Lemon Herbs

Day 10:
- Breakfast: Avocado Toast with Poached Egg
- Lunch: Greek Yogurt Veggie Dip with Crudites
- Dinner: Tofu Stir-Fry with Vegetables

Day 11:

- Breakfast: Mixed Berry Chia Seed Pudding
- Lunch: Kale and Quinoa Salad
- Dinner: Turkey and Vegetable Stir-Fry

Day 12:

- Breakfast: Berry Blast Smoothie
- Lunch: Mediterranean Chickpea Salad

- Dinner: Quinoa and Black Bean Stuffed Bell Peppers

Day 13:

- Breakfast: Dark Chocolate Avocado Mousse
- Lunch: Hummus with Crudites
- Dinner: Eggplant Parmesan

Day 14:

- Breakfast: Banana Oatmeal Cookies
- Lunch: Tomato Basil Soup
- Dinner: Garlic Roasted Brussels Sprouts with Quinoa Pilaf

portion control

- Green Smoothie Bowl: Aim for a serving size of around 1 to 1.5 cups of smoothie base, topped with a variety of fruits, nuts, seeds, and granola, totaling around 300-400 calories.
- Avocado Toast with Poached Egg: One slice of whole-grain bread topped with 1/4 to 1/2 avocado and one poached egg, totaling around 250-350 calories.
- Quinoa Breakfast Bowl: A serving size of cooked quinoa should be around 1/2 to 3/4 cup, topped with fruits, nuts, seeds, and a dollop of yogurt, totaling around 300-400 calories.
- Greek Yogurt Veggie Dip: Aim for a serving size of around 2 tablespoons of dip, paired with a variety of fresh vegetables, totaling around 100-150 calories.
- Baked Sweet Potato Fries: Limit the serving to about 1 small to medium sweet potato per person, totaling around 150-200 calories.
- Hummus with Crudites: Aim for around 2 tablespoons of hummus per serving, accompanied by a variety of raw vegetables, totaling around 150-200 calories.
- Kale and Quinoa Salad: Serve about 1 to 1.5 cups of salad per portion, dressed lightly with vinaigrette, totaling around 250-350 calories.
- Spinach and Strawberry Salad: Aim for about 1 to 1.5 cups of salad per portion, dressed lightly with vinaigrette, totaling around 200-300 calories.
- Mediterranean Chickpea Salad: Serve about 1 to 1.5 cups of salad per portion, dressed with olive oil and lemon juice, totaling around 250-350 calories.
- Lentil Soup: One serving should be around 1 to 1.5 cups, totaling around 250-350 calories.
- Tomato Basil Soup: One serving should be around 1 to 1.5 cups, totaling around 200-300 calories.
- Butternut Squash Soup: One serving should be around 1 to 1.5 cups, totaling around 200-300 calories.
- Lemon Herb Grilled Chicken: Aim for a portion size of about 3-4 ounces of cooked chicken breast per person, totaling around 150-200 calories.
- Baked Salmon with Asparagus: Aim for a portion size of about 3-4 ounces of cooked salmon per person, totaling around 200-250 calories.
- Tofu Stir-Fry with Vegetables: Serve about 1 cup of tofu stir-fry per portion, totaling around 200-300 calories.
- Turkey and Vegetable Stir-Fry: Serve about 1 cup of turkey stir-fry per portion, totaling around 250-350 calories.
- Stuffed Bell Peppers with Quinoa and Black Beans: Aim for one stuffed

- bell pepper per serving, totaling around 300-400 calories.
- Eggplant Parmesan: Aim for a serving size of about 1/6 of a standard eggplant per person, totaling around 300-400 calories.
- Lentil and Vegetable Curry: Serve about 1 to 1.5 cups of curry per portion, accompanied by a portion of rice or quinoa, totaling around 300-400 calories.
- Garlic Roasted Brussels Sprouts: Aim for a serving size of about 1 cup of roasted Brussels sprouts per person, totaling around 100-150 calories.
- Steamed Broccoli with Lemon: Serve about 1 to 1.5 cups of steamed broccoli per portion, totaling around 50-100 calories.

- Quinoa Pilaf: Each portion of cooked quinoa should include between 1/2 and 3/4 cup, or 150–200 calories.
- Mixed Berry Chia Seed Pudding: Aim for a serving size of about 1/2 to 3/4 cup of pudding per person, totaling around 200-250 calories.
- Dark Chocolate Avocado Mousse: Aim for a serving size of about 1/2 cup of mousse per person, totaling around 200-250 calories.
- Banana Oatmeal Cookies: Limit to 1-2 cookies per serving, totaling around 100-150 calories.
- Refreshing Cucumber Mint Water: Enjoy freely as a hydrating beverage with no added calories.

- Homemade Ginger Turmeric Tea: Enjoy freely as a calming beverage with no added calories.

Tips for Meal Preparation and Batch Cooking

Plan Ahead:

- Make time every week to organize your meals. Take into account your diet, timetable, and any ingredients you already have on hand.
- Make a list of recipes you want to prepare for the week and the ingredients required for each meal.

Choose Recipes Wisely:

- Opt for recipes that are simple, versatile, and can be easily scaled up for batch cooking.
- Look for recipes that use similar ingredients to minimize waste and save money.

Invest in Quality Containers:

- Invest in a variety of reusable containers in different sizes to store prepped ingredients and meals.
- Choose containers that are freezer-safe, microwaveable, and stackable for easy storage.

Batch Cooking Basics:

- Decide which day(s) of the week to use for bulk cooking.
- Cook large batches of grains, proteins (such as chicken, tofu, or beans), and vegetables that can be used in multiple meals throughout the week.

Prep Ingredients in Advance:

- Wash, chop, and portion out vegetables, fruits, and herbs ahead of time. Store them in containers or zip-top bags for easy access.
- Pre-cook staples like rice, quinoa, and pasta to save time during the week.

Use Kitchen Gadgets:

- Invest in kitchen gadgets like a slow cooker, Instant Pot, or rice cooker to streamline the cooking process and make batch cooking easier.
- These appliances can help you cook large quantities of food with minimal effort.

Label and Date Everything:

- Label each container with the name of the dish and the date it was prepared to help you keep track of freshness and avoid food waste.
- Use a permanent marker or labels specifically designed for freezer or refrigerator use.

Embrace Freezing:

- Take advantage of your freezer to store batch-cooked meals, soups, stews, and sauces for later use.
- Portion out meals into individual servings before freezing for easier reheating and portion control.

Mix and Match Components:

- Prepare versatile components like roasted vegetables, grilled chicken, or cooked grains that can be mixed and matched to create a variety of meals throughout the week.

Stay Flexible:

- Be flexible with your meal plan and be willing to adjust based on what ingredients are available or on sale.
- Don't be afraid to repurpose leftovers into new dishes to prevent food boredom.

Practice Food Safety:

- Follow proper food safety guidelines when handling and storing perishable foods to prevent foodborne illnesses.

- Perishable items should be refrigerated as soon as possible after cooking.

Enjoy the Process:

- Meal preparation and batch cooking can be a relaxing and enjoyable activity. Put on some music or listen to a podcast while you cook to make the process more enjoyable.

CONCLUSION

In the sumptuous symphony of flavors and nourishment, "Cookbook for Healthy Recipes" transcends mere culinary guidance to become a cherished companion on the journey to wellness. With each turn of its vibrant pages, it whispers secrets of vitality and delight, inviting readers to dance amidst the kaleidoscope of wholesome ingredients and culinary innovation.

As the final chapter draws to a close, it leaves behind a trail of tantalizing aromas and joyful memories, reminding us that true wellness is not just a destination but a harmonious blend of mindful choices and culinary creativity. With every dish crafted with love and intention, this cookbook beckons us to embrace the symphony of tastes and textures that celebrate the abundance of nature.

In the tapestry of life, where health and happiness intertwine, "Cookbook for Healthy Recipes" emerges as a beacon of inspiration, guiding us towards a future where nourishment is not just sustenance but a celebration of vitality. Let its pages be the canvas upon which we paint our culinary dreams, weaving together flavors that nourish the body, delight the senses, and nurture the soul. As we bid farewell to its pages, let us carry its wisdom in our hearts, transforming every meal into a testament to the beauty of living well.